'Chinese Medicine Psychology provides a nice concise survey and elucidation of the classical Chinese understanding of psychological disorders. Part 1 discusses medical principles underlying the *Shén*, its formation, manifestations, roles, functions and maintenance. Part 2 ties in the classical disease patterns from the *Golden Cabinet* with representative formulas. Patho-mechanisms and aetiologies are likewise discussed and modifications are provided. Case studies providing anecdotal real-life formulae round out the text. An excellent reference for students and practitioners alike.'

—*Ross Rosen, author of* Heart Shock: Diagnosis and Treatment of Trauma *with Shen-Hammer and* Classical Chinese Medicine, 23rd and 25th gen. *Quanzhen Longmen Daoist Priest*

'*Chinese Medicine Psychology* is destined to be one of the definitive texts in the field for the diagnosis and treatment of emotional and psychological disorders. Several chapters in part one carefully delineate core concepts from the *Sù wèn*, *Líng Shū*, *Nán Jīng*, *Jīn guì yào lüè* and the work of Zhāng Jǐngyuè (as recorded in the Lèi jīng/Categorized Classic). The second part of the book builds on this understanding to explain the foundations of how classical Chinese medicine views essential aspects of human life, mind and the emotions. In Chapter 9, clinical applications are presented built on material and formulas from Zhāng Zhòngjǐng's *Jīn guì yào lüè /Prescriptions from the Golden Cabinet*, with case histories. As culture is a major influence on psychology, the authors also compare Chinese and Western approaches to psychology, noting similarities and differences.

I highly recommend this text for all practitioners, as *xīn lǐ xué/* psychology is an essential subject that demands clear explanation of terminology, concepts, diagnostics and/or overlays of Western views of the mind and psyche.'

—*Z'ev Rosenberg, LAc*

Chinese Medicine
PSYCHOLOGY

Chinese Medicine
PSYCHOLOGY

A Clinical Guide to Mental and Emotional Wellness

PROFESSOR QU LIFANG (曲丽芳)
and DOCTOR MARY GARVEY (玛丽•嘉伟)

with Doctor Li Weihong (李衛紅)

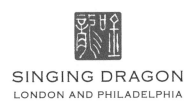

SINGING DRAGON
LONDON AND PHILADELPHIA

Most of the case studies in Chapter 9 have been translated from the Chinese in Professor Qu Lifang's book *Mental and Psychological Diseases: Selected Cases of Ancient Masters* (2015). They are reproduced here with permission. One case is from Qu and Garvey's *Anecdotes of Traditional Chinese Medicine* (2016), also reproduced with permission. Two cases are drawn from the People's Medical Publishing House's *Masters of Chinese Medicine Series* (1960–1980s), and these are referenced accordingly.

First published in 2020
by Singing Dragon
an imprint of Jessica Kingsley Publishers
73 Collier Street
London N1 9BE, UK
and
400 Market Street, Suite 400
Philadelphia, PA 19106, USA

www.singingdragon.com

Library of Congress Cataloging in Publication Data
A CIP catalog record for this book is available from the Library of Congress

British Library Cataloguing in Publication Data
A CIP catalogue record for this book is available from the British Library

ISBN 978 1 78775 276 4
eISBN 978 1 78775 277 1

Printed and bound in the United States

Contents

Preface   9

Part 1: Introduction and Basic Theory **11**

1. What Is Chinese Medicine Psychology?   17
2. Human Life   39
3. The Three Aspects of *Shén*   53
4. Mind and Emotions   71
5. 神明 *Shén Míng*   89
6. Dreams   107
7. Chinese and Western Psychologies   113

Part 2: Diagnosis and Treatment **123**

8. Illness Categories   127
9. Cases   185

Appendix 1: Acupuncture Points   209
Appendix 2: Glossary of Chinese Terms   213
References and Further Reading   229
Index   233

Preface

Chinese medicine is uniquely equipped to assist in the management of mental and emotion-related illnesses, and Chinese medicine psychology is a growing area of clinical practice in China and the West. This book is a professional, clinical practice and learning resource designed to facilitate and promote this important field of healthcare. It provides an introduction and clinical guide for practitioners and students, healthcare professionals and users.

The content is based on both recent and ancient Chinese language, culture and medicine sources. Its theory and practice sections begin with the early medical classics that have guided Chinese medicine practice throughout its history. The discussion applies classical data to the contemporary clinical setting, modern disease categories and individual patient presentations, making these valuable classical resources accessible and relevant for mental health care and illness management today.

Part 1 gives a detailed introduction to the theory of Chinese medicine psychology, including its basis in the early Chinese worldview and classic texts, and modern developments in Chinese medicine psychology theory. It explains previously unavailable material on the generational and ancestral aspects of human mentality, and their context within the natural world and the evolution of human life. Part 2 is a guide to clinical practice based on classical Chinese medicine treatment strategies and formulas, especially those of the *Essential Prescriptions of the Golden Cabinet* (*c.* 220 CE). While these topics will be of interest to many outside the Chinese medicine profession, the authors advise that readers wishing to try Chinese medicine therapies should seek the advice of qualified Chinese medicine practitioners.

The principle authors are experienced Chinese medicine clinicians, researchers and academics. Professor Qu Lifang was the Director of the Golden Cabinet Department at the Shanghai University of Traditional Chinese Medicine until her retirement in 2016. She is a highly sought-after international lecturer who has designed and conducted Chinese medicine courses at the universities of East Finland, Hamburg, Hong Kong, Malta and Sydney, and the international medical university of Malaysia, and training courses in Thailand. Doctor Mary Garvey is a senior lecturer in the Chinese medicine programs at the University of Technology Sydney. Together, Professor Qu and Doctor Garvey have 70 years of clinical, teaching and research experience in the field, and 20 years of co-authored internationally published work. Both are members of the World Federation of Chinese Medicine Societies' Mental Diseases Specialty Committee (Beijing, established 2013).

We gratefully acknowledge the generous assistance and expertise of Doctor Li Weihong, lecturer, clinician and researcher in Chinese medicine at the University of Technology Sydney, who has translated most of the Chapter 9 case studies from Professor Qu's psychology textbook (Qu 2015).

Qu Lifang (曲丽芳) and Mary Garvey (玛丽·嘉伟)
April 2019

PART 1

INTRODUCTION AND BASIC THEORY

In China and the West, clinical evidence is growing for Chinese medicine's effectiveness in assisting the management of many illnesses, including mental and emotional conditions. This book presents an introduction to Chinese medicine psychology and a clinical guide for practitioners.

In Part 1, we present the theories guiding Chinese medicine treatment strategies and the relevant historical and cultural ideas, contexts and terms that underpin them. Chinese medicine terms guide the way in which we view bodily, cognitive and emotional states, and describe the conditions of health and disorder. Accurate terms convey the clinical perspectives and tools that Chinese medicine applies to all kinds of physical and psychological illnesses. Chinese medicine terms are therefore presented throughout using Chinese characters, with pinyin and translations to confirm their meanings and to allow readers to consult and cross-reference to other source texts, textbooks, glossaries and translations. Chapters 1–7 explore Chinese medicine's traditional and contemporary perspectives on human mentality and psychology. These provide a comprehensive explanation of Chinese medicine psychology, and the theories that guide its analysis of mental and emotional disorders. At the conclusion of Part 1 (in Chapter 7), we draw some parallels between Chinese medicine psychology and psychology in the West.

Part 2 applies Chinese medicine theories to the diagnosis and treatment of common psychological illnesses. There are so many psychological categories and diseases that we concentrate on early illness categories and contemporary disease conditions that are common in our clinics today. The discussion presents diagnostic information and treatment strategies that practitioners can readily apply to their patients. It is structured so that we can extend and modify these tools and strategies to interpret and manage a great many mental, emotional, mood and personality disorders, and individualize treatments for specific presentations. The cases in the final chapter help illustrate the application of Chinese medicine theory and practice to the care and management of psychological disorders.

Chinese medicine and Western medicine tend to observe and investigate human life from different perspectives. Generally speaking, for example, Chinese medicine does not separate a person's illness experiences into psychological or physical categories. Even so, the Chinese medicine classics contain a great deal of information on what we nowadays call 'psychology.' Their many references to human mentality reveal detailed perspectives that remain relevant for practice in the present day.

Its historical records show that Chinese medicine investigated and described human life from ancient times. It saw the living body as 'a cosmos, combining cognitive ingredients, social ideals, physical data, and sensual self-awareness' (Lloyd and Sivin 2002, p.218). Classical doctrines that describe early perspectives form the general principles for Traditional Chinese Medicine (TCM) theory and practice today. TCM's general principles and basic theories apply to all areas of clinical practice, and our presentation of them in Part 1 emphasizes those aspects most relevant for the understanding, diagnosis and treatment of psychological diseases. The relationships and dynamics of the living human body, its source and beginning, its organ systems and *qì* substances, the three levels of *shén*-spirit/mind, the emotions and personality, are central features of TCM's approach to psychology. As a construct of the 1950s and 1960s, 'TCM' is the current Chinese medicine orthodoxy. In this book, 'TCM' therefore refers to modern Chinese medicine, and 'Chinese medicine' to the whole of Chinese medicine, including its classic texts and historical currents.

In philosophy and medicine, the Chinese notion of 气 *qì* (function, influence, very fine substance) bridges the accepted distinctions between matter and energy, body and mind. According to ancient cosmology, all phenomena throughout the universe are interrelated because they arise from a single point, the 'great ultimate' (太极 *tài jí*), and share this one source.[1]

Thus, from at least the time of the *Zhuāng Zǐ*[2] (late 4th century BCE), Chinese philosophy emphasized the idea of the 'one *qì* running through heaven and earth,' through all immaterial and material, insubstantial and substantial things. Consequently, the concept of 气 *qì* embraces the inter-convertibility of matter and energy, and therefore, in Chinese medicine the body and mind are not just closely linked. Similarly, and while signaling the psychological aspects of human life, the term 神 *shén* (spirit/mind) also challenges the idea that the body and mind are separate entities.

Chinese medicine's earliest classic text is the *Yellow Emperor's Inner Canon*[3] (*c.* 100 BCE), hereafter the *Inner Canon*. Its authors discussed all manner of physiological and functional life activities, including thinking, intuition, emotions, sensations and dreaming. While today we consider all these activities mental rather than physical, the concepts of 气 *qì* and 神 *shén* contest the distinction. The perspectives we find in the *Inner Canon* are first explained in the *Book of Changes*[4] (from *c.* 700 BCE), one of China's most ancient and famous classics. Early Chinese philosophy strongly influenced the development of China's early life sciences. In the *Book of Changes*, and in both philosophy and medicine, the constant fluidity of change, the transformations of *qì* and the inter-relatedness of all things, are described by the inter-dependency and inter-transformation of *yīn* and *yáng*.[5] *Yīn–yáng* is

---

1   This idea is known as '*qì* monism' or 'monism' (一元论 *yī yuán lùn*): the primary or primordial *qì* is the basis of all phenomena in the universe. The law (道 *dào*) of the universe starts from nothingness (无极 *wú jí*, without time or space). From nothingness comes 'the one' (太极 *tài jí*), the primordial *qì* (混元气 *hùn yuán qì*), also called 'chaos *qì*' (混沌气 *hùn dùn qì*). Everything comes from this one *qì*. Therefore, the concept of 气 *qì* encompasses energy and function, and the smallest particles of matter, throughout the universe

2   《莊子》 *Zhuāngzǐ* is an ancient Chinese collection of fables; attributed to Zhuāng Zǐ ('Master Zhuang,' *c.* 369–286 BCE, it is one of the foundational texts of Daoism

3   《黄帝内经》 *Huáng dì nèi jīng*: the *Inner Canon* is in two parts, the 素问 *Sù wèn* (*Elementary Questions*), and the 灵枢 *Líng shū* (*Divine Pivot*), each with 81 treatises

4   《易经》 *Yì jīng*

5   阴阳 *yīn yáng* (陰陽 are the traditional, complex characters)

another important idea for TCM and we take a closer look at it in Chapter 1.

In the *Inner Canon*, the 'body form and spirit/mind' (形神 *xíng shén*) concept is built on the functioning inter-relatedness of material and energetic resources. The *shén*-spirit/mind depends on the living body for its existence. The body provides its dwelling place, and the body's transformation and movement of *qì*, blood and essence supply the material basis for *shén qì* activities and influences. The *shén* for its part guides the body's *qì* movements, transformations and materializations. The *shén*'s directing influences shape the body form, its physiological process-events, its active (*yáng*) and structured (*yīn*) states. As well as guiding our physical and physiological features, the *shén* is the principle force that conditions our character and personality.

Every human life has attributes and abilities derived from many generations of human evolution, and depending on our inherited allotment, each has certain potentials and resources for developing those abilities. The interactions between inherited and acquired resources have far-reaching implications for our physical, mental, emotional and psychological development. These ideas are fundamental for TCM theories of life, health and illness, and help explain the importance it places on self-cultivation to maintain physical and mental health.

The 神 *shén*-spirit/mind consists of both inherited (prenatal) and acquired (postnatal) influences, and we analyze these influences and conditions according to three levels or developmental stages of human mentality:

- The 'root *shén*' (本神 *běn shén*), the accumulation of experiences that have been acquired by all our ancestors over millions of years of evolution.

- The 'initiating *shén*' (元神 *yuán shén*), the first impetus of life and carrier of the abilities, potentials and instinctual functions of the root *shén*.

- The 'acquired *shén*' (识神 *shì shén*), our cognitive capacity derived from the initiating *shén* and moulded by the activities of our postnatal life.

The *Inner Canon* does not specifically differentiate between the prenatal and postnatal *shén*. But from at least the Tang dynasty (618–907 CE), Daoist meditators placed great importance on the initiating *shén* as a kind of spiritual consciousness. Because it exists before birth, it was thought to be part of the primal or 'initiating *qì*' (元气 *yuán qì*) that pervades the whole universe. The postnatal (acquired) *shén*, which consists of the senses, feelings, thoughts and perceptions we experience during our lifetime, was considered ordinary consciousness. Prenatal and postnatal features of the *shén* are recorded in the medical literature from the Song dynasty (960–1278), and were drawn from Daoist and Buddhist sources where the distinction was an important idea for self-cultivation practices.

The three levels or aspects of *shén* provide a comprehensive explanation of the characteristics and abilities of human psychology. TCM analyzes the third level, the acquired *shén*, using its 'mind theory' (神志学说 *shén zhì xué shuō*). *Shén zhì* theory is essential for interpreting the clinical manifestations of psychological disorder in clinical practice. Its origins are found in the *Inner Canon.*

Chapter 1

What Is Chinese Medicine Psychology?

For the study of Chinese medicine psychology, it is useful to keep in mind the distinction between Western 'psychology'[6] and early Chinese 'psychological thought.'[7] 'Chinese psychological thought' was the term used by Harold Roth (1991) for China's early conceptions of human mentality. Similarly, we use it here as a broad term for the discipline's early conceptions of human life and mentality, and to distinguish them from recent developments in Western and TCM psychology. Psychology, the 100-year-old field that developed initially in Europe, is 'without parallels in ancient China' (Roth 1991), despite the fact that Western and TCM psychology have some surprising connections, which we briefly explore in Chapter 7.

To understand Chinese medicine psychological thought and TCM psychology we must first understand key ideas, terms and theories relevant to the field. The meaning of Chinese medicine terms, even very familiar ones such as 气 *qì*, the spirit/mind (神 *shén*), the heart (心 *xīn*) and emotions (情 *qíng*), are best understood in their historical, cultural and textual contexts. For example, 神 *shén* has accumulated various connotations over thousands of years and its meaning can change according to its context in philosophical and religious texts, cultural traditions and common language. So, we begin with some

---

6   心理学 *xīnlǐ xué*
7   心理思想 *xīnlǐ sīxiǎng*

history and background to explain China's early worldview and its perspectives on human life and mentality.

Early Chinese worldview

In Chapter 42 of the *Classic of the Law and Its Power*[8] (*c.* 460 BCE), all things arise at the intersection of heaven and earth. This includes human life, and the potentials of each individual human life arise at the moment of conception. At conception, the meeting of the sperm and ovum is an individual instance of the intersection of heaven and earth, *yáng* and *yīn*. Early Chinese medicine's adoption of philosophical concepts such as *qì* and *yīn–yáng*, was part of the deep cultural shift that began in China towards the end of the Warring States period (475–221 BCE) and gradually replaced demonic and ancestral explanations with a more nature-based worldview.

Because human life is a kind of natural phenomenon, its vitality and bioenergy are part of the power of nature. Human life, therefore, must also follow the *dào* (道) and its fundamental natural law, *yīn* and *yáng*. The authors of the *Inner Canon* (*c.* 100 BCE) use *yīn–yáng* extensively to explain the connections between nature and human life. In the *Inner Canon*, the *Elementary Questions* Treatises 3 and 5,[9] for example, discuss the comprehensiveness of *yīn–yáng* for cosmology, the environment, human physiology, diet, emotions, illness, aging and so on.

Even before the *Classic of the Law and Its Power*, it was the *Book of Changes* (from *c.* 700 BCE) that introduced the relational and contingent framework of *yīn–yáng* natural law. The worldview of the *Changes* was developed by careful and detailed observation and contemplation of nature's organic relationships over long periods of time. Its interpretations deeply influenced all of China's philosophical and proto-scientific traditions, including Chinese medicine.

---

8   《道德经》 *Dào dé jīng*, also known as the 《老子》 *Lǎo Zǐ*, 'Old Master'. Lǎo Zǐ (*c.* 6th century BCE) is considered the founder of philosophical Daoism ('cosmic law' and the 'way'), and is said to be the author of the *Dào dé jīng*

9   Treatise 3: 生气通天伦 *Shēng qì tōng tiān lún* ('Discourse on How the Generative *Qì* Communicates with Heaven [the Universe]'), and Treatise 5: 阴阳应象大论 *Yīn yáng yīng xiàng dà lùn* ('Comprehensive Discourse on Phenomena Corresponding to Yīn and Yáng')

Historically, Chinese medicine texts frequently acknowledge the importance of the *Book of Changes* for medicine. In the Tang dynasty (618–907), Sūn Sīmiǎo said: 'If you don't understand the *Book of Changes*, you cannot talk about medicine,'[10] and in 1624, Zhāng Jièbīn said:

> Medicine and the *Changes* are the same. [This is because] Nature/ heaven and human beings conform to the same laws, namely, the principles of *yīn–yáng*. And though medical practice is complicated, we can use *yīn–yáng* to summarize and analyze all its permutations.[11]

The *Book of Changes'* notions of being (ontology) and knowing (epistemology) connect all material and immaterial phenomena. Its *yīn–yáng* natural law, and '*dào*–phenomenon–entity'[12] cosmology were important influences on early Chinese thinking. This view of reality and being led Chinese medical investigations to focus on function and process, the emergent manifestations of life and the living body, more so than its material structures.

The *dào*–phenomenon–entity triad stands for 'abstract principles,' 'emergent manifestations' and 'concrete objects,' respectively. According to the *Changes* and its Great Commentary,[13] the *dào* (道 the 'law,' the 'way') is before space and time. It is not visible and without substance. The *qì* (器 concrete and material things) are visible. They occupy space and time because they occur after the interactions of *yīn–yáng* natural law and have substance and shape. Consequently, the binome 道器 *dào qì* (cosmic law and material entity) is an expression for the relationship between abstract and concrete, the power of natural law and the resulting objects and entities. 象 *Xiàng*-phenomena are manifestations and the bridge linking invisible abstract potentials (道) and concrete things (器). The *xiàng* can be observed at the point of emergence between the *dào* and *qì* aspects of reality. *Xiàng*-manifestations are the observable indications of *yīn–yáng* natural law (Zhang 2002).

All phenomena and entities in the universe, including human beings, have their own point in space and time. Therefore, they must conform

---

10 孙思邈：'不知易，不足以言太医。Sūn Sīmiǎo: *'Bù zhī yì, bù zú yǐ yán tài yī'*
11 张介宾：'医易相同。天人一理也，一此阴阳也。医道虽繁，而可一言以 蔽之者，曰：阴阳而已。Zhāng Jièbīn: *'Yī yì xiāng tóng. Tiān rén yī lǐ yě, yī cǐ yīn yáng yě. Yī dào suī fán, ér kè yī yán yǐ bì zhī zhě, yuē: Yīn yáng ér yǐ'*
12 道象器 *dào xiàng qì*
13 《大傳》 *Dà Zhuán* (c. 300 BCE)

with the processes of space and time in their coming and going, life and death. In the *Book of Changes*, this endless succession and continuous generation and coming to being is called *The Changes*.[14] It explains that, 'What cannot be measured by *yīn–yáng* are called *shén* [the power of nature],' and 'When entity and substance appear and are clearly visible this is *míng* [clarity].'[15] The *Elementary Questions* Treatise 5 draws on *The Changes* when it says that:

> *Yīn* and *yáng* are the law (道) of heaven and earth, the principles governing all things, the parents of all changes and transformations, the origin of birth and death, the place of *shén* brightness (神明 *shén míng*).[16]

Guided by *The Changes'* onto-epistemic, Chinese medical methods are characterized by a functional perspective based on observable phenomena. Chinese medicine explores human life phenomena, including its visceral (脏/藏 *zàng*) functions and manifestations (藏 象 *zàng xiàng*). In fact, today this is TCM's 'visceral manifestations theory,'[17] which is considered the cornerstone of Chinese diagnostic thinking and medical practice (Qu and Garvey 2008).

Human nature

In China, questions concerning the human mind were first recorded in the Warring States period (475–221 BCE), and were associated with debates about 'human nature' (性 *xìng*). The meaning of 性 *xìng* included instincts, and in the *Xúnzǐ*[18] (c. 238 BCE), the Confucian philosopher Master Xun observed that it is human nature to want to eat when hungry, to get warm when feeling cold and to rest after labor. From earliest times, the Chinese considered human instincts, abilities and senses to be a part of human nature, and so were emotions and talents. Line 3 of the *Xúnzǐ* 22 'On the Rectification of Terms' says:

---

14 《易经》：生生之为易 *Yì jīng: Shēng shēng zhī wèi yì*

15 《易经》：阴阳不测谓之神 *Yì jīng: Yīn yáng bù cè wèi zhī shén*; and 《内经知 要》李中梓：品物流行谓之明。*Nèi jīng zhī yào* (by *Lǐ Zhōngzǐ* 1588–1655): *Pǐn wù liú xíng wèi. zhī míng*

16 《素问·阴阳应象大论》：阴阳者，天地之道也，万物之纲纪，变化之父 母，生杀之本使，神明之府也。*Sù wèn, Yīn yáng yīng xiàng dà lùn: Yīn yáng zhě, tiān dì zhī dào yě, wàn wù zhī gāng jì, biàn huà zhī fù mǔ, shēng shā zhī běn shǐ, shén míng zhī fǔ yě*

17 藏象学说 *zàng xiàng xué shuō*

18 荀子 *Xúnzǐ*, 'Master Xun' (c. 312–230 BCE)

'The liking, disliking, joy, anger, grief and happiness of human nature are what is meant by emotions.' Line 2 states that, 'Whereby life is as it is (性 *xìng*), is called nature (天 *tiān*)' (Geaney 2002; Zhang 2002).

According to Daoism, the inherent characteristics that are our 'root nature' (本性 *běn xìng*) come from the natural world (天 *tiān* 'heaven'). Therefore, the natural world/heaven is within the nature (性) of every human life. This 'root nature' (本性 *běn xìng*) of human life has two aspects. One is 'biological instincts' (本能 *běn néng*), and the other is the instincts of the 'root *shén*' (本神 *běn shén*).

本性 **Běn xìng** (our root nature) has two aspects:

本神 *Běn shén* (miraculous spirit/mind abilities and functions)

本能 *Běn néng* (biological abilities and functions).

Běn néng means our unlearned biological functions and capabilities, and *běn shén* means the innate nature of our *shén*-spirit/mind, our human qualities, character, behavior and personality traits. We look at the relationship between the natural world and human life in more detail in the next chapter.

The 'mind'

TCM today identifies the 神 *shén* with human conscious awareness, the mind. The translation of *shén* as 'mind' will facilitate our exploration of TCM psychology; however, most of its translations—'mind,' 'psyche' and 'spirit' for instance—are not helpful to correctly understand Chinese medical and psychological concepts. We therefore retain the term *shén* to distinguish Chinese and Western psychological discourses, and to avoid the dichotomous body and mind connotations and religious ideas carried by English translations. The extended meanings of *shén* presented here inform our analysis of mental and emotional traits and patterns, and our interpretations of the *shén*'s clinical manifestations.

Originally, 神 *shén* was used to describe the ubiquitous and mysterious power of nature. In everyday language it referred to gods and divinities. In the *Inner Canon*, *shén* is a special kind of *qì* (气) that has these same numinous qualities producing normal life activities. In the *Inner Canon*, *shén* is the difference between a lifeless body and a living person—it is what transforms a body into a complex, living person: it is the phenomenon of sentient life.

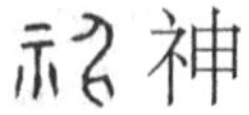

示己 神

*Figure 1.1: Early pictograph and modern
character for the 神 shén-spirit/mind*

The early Chinese pictograph for *shén* is shown on the left, and the modern character (神) on the right is shown for comparison. Both have two parts. The old form for the radical on the left (礻) was 示 *shì*, which meant 'show' and 'display,' and represented sacrificial offerings on an 'altar.' On the right is an image of a person kneeling with respect. The early form of the character reflects the veneration the Chinese people felt for the 'power of nature,' the 天神 *tiān shén*.

Another analysis of the character (Wieger 1965) explains that the upper part of 示 (二) can represent 'heaven and earth,' but is also an early form of 上 *shàng*-above, meaning 'the heavens.' The lower part shows the three types of illumination, the sun, moon and stars, that hang from the heavens. The sun, moon and stars are the 'three lights' (三光 *sān guāng*), the radiance of heaven/nature that illuminates human life on earth. The luminescence of the sun, moon and stars corresponds to the 'three treasures' (三宝 *sān bǎo*) of an individual human life, their 'essence *qì* and *shén*' (精气神 *jīng qì shén*). The correspondence indicates that the three treasures have inherited ancestral qualities that are connected to the radiant power of nature (天神 *tiān shén*).

The ancient Chinese deeply understood the 'union of nature and human life.'[19] They understood that protecting and respecting nature was the same as protecting and respecting oneself. The *Inner Canon* reiterates these ideas, such as in the *Elementary Questions* Treatise 74, where it says, 'The great arrangements of heaven and earth, this is what human life (人神 *rén shén*) corresponds to.'[20] To understand the significance of the term *shén* is to understand human life as a special manifestation of nature. We discuss the relationship between nature (天神 *tiān shén*) and human life (人神 *rén shén*) in more detail in Chapter 3.

Translations of ancient texts tend to use 'mind' for the term 心 *xīn* (the 'heart'). In the *Xúnzǐ*, the heart-mind (心) coordinated and interpreted the body's sensory perceptions. The *Xúnzǐ* Section 22

---

19 天人合一 *tiān rén hé yī*
20 《素问·至真要大论》：天地之大纪，人神之通应也。*Sù wèn, Zhì zhēn yào dà lùn: 'Tiān dì zhī dà jì, rén shén zhī tōng yìng yě'*

explains that the mind (心) encounters the outside world directly via the five senses. The heart-mind's 'impressions' include its ability to recognize and assess the information we perceive, and the early texts consistently associate clear perceptions with mental brightness and intelligence. In the *Inner Canon*, sensory perceptions are also closely tied to mentality.

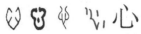

Figure 1.2: Early pictographs and modern character for the 心 xīn-heart

The first three images on the left are early pictographs for the character 心 *xīn*-heart. Interestingly, they all depict anatomical features, the chambers of the heart for instance. The fourth image is from the *Book of Rites*[21] and reflects a shift in meaning when, from the Warring states period (475–221 BCE), the heart is aligned with the *shén*, our cognitive functions and mental and emotional life. The *Inner Canon* uses the term heart (心) to signify both the *yīn* visceral system and the 'mind.'

The fifth image is the modern character and of all the characters for Chinese medicine's internal organs, only the heart (心 *xīn*) is written without the flesh radical.[22] The character consists of three dots over the main central stroke, which is open at the top like a container. The character shows that of the three dots, only the middle one is kept. This alludes to the heart's memory function: the heart (the main central stroke) only selects on balance the things to keep and store. The dots represent our everyday experiences and those on the left and right are not selected to be held in the heart. Because they are off to the sides, they are like 'positive and negative,' 'good and bad,' 'happy and sad' experiences, the mental and emotional extremes that should not be kept in the heart.

The heart radical (忄) is seen in many words for emotional states[23] and illustrates a similar idea. But rather than a container, the radical's main central stroke is vertical and straight and means 'even.' The stroke is upright and neutral; it is flexible but quickly returns to its

---

21 《礼记》 *Lǐ jì* (Warring States period, exact dates unknown)

22 The flesh radical 月 *ròu* is seen for example in 肺 *fèi* (lung), 肝 *gān* (liver), 肾 *shèn* (kidney) and 脾 *pí* (spleen), but not in 心 *xīn* (heart)

23 For example, in words such as 情 *qíng* (love), 怡 *yí* (joy), 忧 *yōu* (worry), 悚 *sǒng* (frightened), 悦 *yuè* (happiness) and 恼 *nǎo* (anger)

even and balanced position. Emotions affect our *qì* influences and their movement: for example, anger causes the *qì* to rise, and fear causes it to descend; joy slows the *qì*, and sadness weakens the *qì*. While emotional responses are a normal part of life, overly strong and prolonged emotions disrupt the *qì* and can lead to emotional disorder. Eventually they injure the internal viscera and can shorten a person's life. The heart radical illustrates that our feelings and moods ought to remain even and neutral. In this way, we follow our natural, instinctual desire for a peaceful inner life.

The *Inner Canon* often uses another word for 'mind': 志 *zhì*. It is a general term for the 'emotions' and 'temperament,' the 'mind,' 'memory' and 'will,' but unlike the 心 *xīn*-heart, all the meanings for 志 *zhì* refer to non-physical features. For example, the *Inner Canon* explains the early medical perspectives of the five emotions or 'five intents' (五志 *wǔ zhì*), sometimes called the 'five minds'—joy, anger, sadness, pensiveness and fear. In the 12th and 13th centuries, the relationships between our *qì* and our emotional responses were further elaborated on when the 'five minds' were extended to the 'seven emotions' (七情 *qī qíng*) by including worry and fright. Significant emotional experiences become part of our memory/mind (志 *zhì*) and we remember them our whole life. Another name for the *zhì*-mind/memory is 情志 *qíng zhì*.

Thus, the English word 'mind' is often used to translate several Chinese terms—心 *xīn*, 神 *shén*, 心神 *xīn shén*, 志 *zhì*, and 神志 *shén zhì* (see Chapter 4). 'Emotions' is the usual translation for 情 *qíng*, 志 *zhì*, and 情志 *qíng zhì*, although for 志 *zhì* we should remember that its meaning encompasses disposition, temperament, mind, memory, will, intelligence and ambition,[24] features that are closely related to the kidney visceral system.

There is one more term to mention here. In the *Inner Canon*, 精神 *jīng shén* means 'essence' and 'mental vitality.' During the Warring States period (475–221 BCE), 精 *jīng*-essence meant 'pure and quintessential.' In Chinese medicine, *jīng*-essence became the term for the material basis of human life and its 神气 *shén qì*. While 神 *shén* referred to the vitality and phenomena of life, *jīng*-essence was

---

24 For accuracy's sake, we note that each of these qualities has their own Chinese term: 性情 *xìng qíng* ('disposition'), 性格 *xìng gé* ('temperament'), 智力 *zhì lì* ('mind'), 记忆 *jì yì* ('memory'), 意志 *yì zhì* ('will'), 智慧 *zhì huì* ('intelligence') and 志向 *zhì xiàng* ('ambition')

the basis of life, and it was the *shén* that guided the materialization of *qì* influences and shaped the body form. We return to this important concept, the *jīng shén*, when we look at the origin of human life in Chapter 2.

Early psychological disorders

In general, the *Inner Canon* does not draw a very distinct line between mental and physical resources and manifestations, and tends to discuss illness in ways that are consistent with a unified view of the body and mind. Yet there are instances where it clearly identifies mental features and conditions, such as the three severe *shén* disorders 'insanity-withdrawal' (癲 *diān*), 'mania' (狂 *kuáng*), and 'epilepsy' (癇 *xián*). In the *Inner Canon*, 癲狂 *diān kuáng* is an obvious example of mental illness involving incoherent behavior, distorted perceptions and hallucinations, dulled responses and cognitive deterioration. Insanity and mania correspond to contemporary psychiatric illnesses such as schizophrenia and bi-polar disorders, while today epilepsy (癇 *xián*) is considered a neurological disorder.

Possession

Possession by ghosts and demons was the cause of madness and epilepsy in ancient China, and for a long time, 狂 *kuáng*-mania and 癇 *xián*-epilepsy were sometimes described as 'wind' (风 *fēng*) disorders.[25] But by the time of the compilation of the *Inner Canon* in the Han dynasty (206 BCE–220 CE), a more naturalist empiricism was replacing magical and demonic accounts, and there it describes *diān kuáng* as severe *shén* disorders caused by various pathogenic states. Pathogenic states arose due to disharmony between *yīn* and *yáng*, *qì* and blood, repletion and depletion. Over time, Chinese physicians began to attribute madness or possession-like symptoms to the sudden blocking of the 'heart aperture' (心窍 *xīn qìao*) by 'phlegm' (痰 *tán*).[26] From about the 14th century, the symptoms of madness were also associated with phlegm fire pathogenic factors.

---

25 Such as 'wind mania' (风狂 *fēng kuáng*), or 'heart wind' (心风 *xīn fēng*)

26 痰迷心窍 *tán mí xīn qìao*, an illness pattern

Chinese medicine's analysis of *shén* disorders begins in the Eastern Han (25–220 CE) with the *Canon of Difficult Issues*[27] and the *Essential Prescriptions of the Golden Cabinet*.[28] In the *Canon of Difficult Issues*, Issue 20, a doubling of *yáng* or *yīn* leads to insanity—mania (狂 *kuáng*) in the case of excess *yáng*, and withdrawal-insanity (癫 *diān*) if the *yīn* is excess.[29] Issues 20 and 59 explain that:

> A doubling of the *yáng* [results in] mania; a doubling of the *yīn* [results in] insanity-withdrawal. When the *yáng* are lost, one sees demons; when the yin are lost, one's eyes turn blind… During the initial development of mania (狂 *kuáng*), one rests only rarely and does not feel hungry. One will speak of oneself as occupying a lofty, exemplary position. One will point out one's special wisdom, and one will behave in an arrogant and haughty way. One will laugh—and find joy in singing and making music—without reason, and one will walk around heedlessly without break. During the initial development of insanity-withdrawal (癫 *diān*), one's thoughts are unhappy. One lies down and stares straight ahead. The pulses of *yīn* and the *yáng* are full in all three positions.

While the *Canon of Difficult Issues* records the observable manifestations of *yīn–yáng* repletion states, in the *Golden Cabinet*, Zhāng Zhòngjǐng[30] (150–219 CE) notes how *diān kuáng* can occur due to depletions. Line 11.12 describes a type of *shén* disorder where there is 'evil crying,' a severe emotional disturbance with no apparent reason. Here Zhāng introduces the '*hún–pò* wandering' disorder, illustrates the impact of disruption to the *jīng shén* relationship, and links its pathogenesis with depleted blood and *qì*.[31]

> When evil crying disquiets the *hún* and *pò*, blood and *qì* are scant. Scantiness of blood and *qì* is associated with the heart. The patient is fearful, closes their eyes and desires to sleep, experiences dreaming and sleepwalking [caused by] separated and dispersed *jīng shén*, and frenetic wandering of the *hún* and *pò*. Debilitation of *yīn qì* causes *diān*-withdrawal; debilitation of *yáng qì* causes *kuáng*-mania.

27　《难经》 *Nán jīng, c.* 100 CE
28　《金匮要略》 *Jīn guì yào lüè*, originally *c.* 220 CE
29　重阳者狂，重阴者癫。 *Chóng yáng zhě kuáng, chòng yīn zhě diān*
30　张仲景 Zhāng Zhòngjǐng
31　血气少也 *Xuè qì shǎo yě*

Illness categories with explicit connotations of mental disorder began to appear in the Chinese medicine literature in the latter part of the Ming dynasty (1368–1644). In the meantime, Chinese physicians were mostly content to expand upon the illness categories and pathomechanisms described in the early classics. The *Inner Canon* had established the emotions as 'inner causes' of illness, in contrast to the 'external causes,' the climatic factors. Later masters such as Líu Wánsù[32] (*c.* 1120–1200) argued that generally, *diān* was associated more with joy, and *kuáng* with anger, and that all five emotions tended to generate internal heat. Zhū Dānxī[33] (1281–1358) took up this idea, incorporating the Neo-Confucian view that emotions were actually rooted in the inner fire of human life and its conscious awareness.

Hallucinations

Today, when the patient's speech, behavior, cognitive and emotional responses are disconnected from reality, this is psychosis. In the Ming dynasty, Lǐ Tǐng (dates unknown)[34] defined the disorder in terms of hallucinations and abnormal behavior. In the 'Withdrawal and Mania' section of his *Introduction to Medicine*, Lǐ Yán said: 'All looking, hearing, speaking and actions are abnormal, this is *xié suì*.'[35]

In the Han dynasty dictionary, *Explaining and Analysing Characters* (121 CE),[36] the entry for 邪 *xié* is 'abnormal,' and 祟 *suì* means '*shén* disaster.' Together in 邪祟病 *xié suì bìng* the term refers to severe *shén* disorders, as if the person is possessed. In severe disorders, the senses convey false and distorted sensations that are unrelated to an actual source: hallucinations. Hallucinations may be seen, heard, smelt or tasted. They may be tactile, such as pain, itching or crawling sensations under the skin, or sensations of heat or cold that are unrelated to environmental or physiological conditions.

Although the *Inner Canon* does not use the term *xié suì* (邪祟), it mentions 'human life' (人神 *rén shén*) in its description of the illness

---

32 刘完素 Líu Wánsù

33 朱丹溪 Zhū Dānxī

34 李梴 Lǐ Yán (active during the Ming dynasty's Jia Jing 嘉靖 to Wan Li 万历 periods, 1522–1566 to 1573–1620)

35 《医学入门·癫狂》: 视听言动俱妄者，谓之邪祟。 *Yī xué rù mén, 'Diān kuáng': 'Shì tīng yán dòng jù wàng zhě, wèi zhī xié suì'*

36 《说文解字》 *Shuō wén jiě zì*, written by 许慎 Xǔ Shèn (*c.* 58–147)

and its circumstances. In the *Elementary Questions* Treatise 73, Huáng Dì says that if the person's *qì* is depleted and this combines with an insufficiency of heaven *qì*, these are the conditions where:

> *Rén shén* fails to keep its normal position, *shén* light can no longer gather, evil ghosts can disturb the person, they are bewitched, lost, and may die.[37]

In Treatise 73, '*rén shén* failure to keep its position' means there is a failure to protect the inner root of human life. When the inner root is not protected, '*shén* light' (神光 *shén guāng*) cannot gather and concentrate, causing functional and mental derangement. The person easily succumbs to pathogenic influences, mental disturbances, hallucinations, and even death.

Treatise 73 describes five kinds of failure to protect the inner root, one for each of the *yīn* viscera. All involve some form of 'heavenly *qì* depletion' (天虚 *tiān xū*) combined with human life *qì* depletion, conditions that cause the *shén* to wander and lose its position. In the *Inner Canon* these conditions result in five kinds of *shén* mis-position and loss of enlightenment, called 'corpse ghost disturbances' (尸厥 *shī jué*). In one example, when the year of fire is insufficient, black corpse ghosts can appear because when the heart is weakened the kidney overcomes it, and black is the color that corresponds to the kidney.

In the *Inner Canon*, the heart holds the office of monarch. The heart lodges the *shén* and for normal psychological development, *shén* brightness accrues from orderly heart-*shén* activities. Let's say, for example, that too much grief or worry consumes heart blood and damages the heart, and then the person experiences strong fear so that sweating comes from the heart. In difficult circumstances such as this, the *shén* fails to keep its normal position, *shén* light cannot gather and cognitive dysfunction arises. Treatise 73 explains that if at the same time there is heavenly deficiency (天虚), this state is called the 'three vacuities' (三虚 *sān xū*). *Tiān xū* means there is insufficient governance of the heart by heaven, an idea that comes from the 'five circuits and six *qì*' and 'inner root' theories discussed below in Chapter 2.

When the three vacuities are present (heavenly deficiency, visceral depletion and strong fear that causes sweating), these conditions are

---

37   《素问·本病论》：**人神**失守，**神光**不聚，邪鬼干人，致人妖亡。 *Sù wèn, Běn bìng lùn*: '**Rén shén** shī shǒu, **shén guāng** bù jù, xié guǐ gàn rén, zhì rén yāo wáng'

disastrous for the *shén*, and evil *qì* prevails. The *Elementary Questions* warns that the person is lost and may die suddenly. Therefore, the *Inner Canon* often says, 'With *shén*, life flourishes; without *shén*, life perishes' (this particular quote is from the *Elementary Questions* Treatise 23).

The 'mind category'

Wáng Kěntáng[38] (1549–1613) was another influential scholar/physician in the late Ming. He and some of his contemporaries gathered together previously scattered references to mental and emotional disorders to provide a systematic survey of the topic. By recording over a dozen mental illness terms under a category called 'mind disorders' (神志病 *shén zhì bìng*), his *Standards of Patterns and Treatments*[39] established a new category of illnesses called the '*shén zhì* category.'[40]

Wáng Kěntáng's *shén zhì* category includes disorders such as 'insanity-withdrawal' (癫 *diān*), 'mania' (狂 *kuáng*), 'epilepsy' (痫 *xián*), the 'seven emotions' (七情 *qī qíng*), 'depletion vexation' (虚烦 *xū fán*), 'agitation' (躁 *zào*), 'fright' (惊 *jīng*) and 'heart palpitations' (心悸 *xīn jì*). He stresses the importance and authority of the classic texts over later medical discourses, and quotes extensively from the *Inner Canon*, *Canon of Difficult Issues*, *Pulse Classic*,[41] *Essential Prescriptions of the Golden Cabinet*, and the *Prescriptions Worth a Thousand Gold*.[42] Even though Wáng Kěntáng's new *shén zhì* category did not seem to make a major impact on Ming and Qing dynasty medical discourses, in retrospect it was a significant development for Chinese medicine psychological thinking.

Also in the late Ming, Zhāng Jièbīn[43] (1563–1640) proposed a category of 'emotional disorders' (情志病 *qíng zhì bìng*) in his famous annotations on the *Inner Canon*, the *Classified Classic*.[44] So it was that from around this time the terms 'emotional states' (情志 *qíng zhì*) and

---

38 王肯堂 Wáng Kěntáng
39 《证治准绳》 *Zhèng zhì zhǔn shéng* (1602)
40 神志门 *shén zhì mén*
41 《脉经》 *Mài jīng* (*c.* 280 CE), by 王叔和 Wáng Shūhé (210–280)
42 《千金要方》 *Qiān jīn yào fāng* (680 CE), by Sun Simiao (581–682)
43 张介宾 Zhāng Jièbīn (also known as, 张景岳 Zhāng Jǐngyuè)
44 《类经》 *Lèi jīng* (1624)

'mental states' (神志 *shén zhì*) entered the Chinese medicine lexicon (Chiu 1986).

Early treatment strategies

According to its historical archive, Chinese medicine generally attributed psychological illness to excess or prolonged mental or emotional states. However, it also clearly recognized the importance of social and personal conditions, as well as inherited, acquired, nutritional and illness factors and other pathogenic factors. From earliest times, Chinese notions of health are contiguous with a person's life habits and practices, and a person's self-cultivation is continuous with their family, social, professional and political relations, activities and circumstances (Farquhar 1994; Sivin 1987).

Diagnosis was based on the observed manifestations of disturbance affecting the patient's *qì* influences and substances, and treatments were designed to rectify the disruptions identified. Treatments mostly took the form of medicinal prescriptions, although the archive shows that decocted medicinal preparations were not the only approach to the management of psychological illness.

Many Ming dynasty (1368–1644) doctors believed that mental and emotional illnesses were more difficult to treat than other types of illness. The general consensus was that they could not be cured unless the patient cultivated contentment and lack of concern for success or failure, good or bad. Zhāng Jièbīn, for example, felt that women's emotional illnesses could be relieved only when their wishes were fulfilled, while men could not be cured unless they knew 'when to yield and when not to,' or they had cultivated 'a detached mind and supreme wisdom' (Chen 2014). Not only Chinese medicine prescriptions and the doctor's skill, but also the patient's character and self-awareness, were thought to be decisive for recovery. We return to the topic of lifestyle and self-cultivation in Chapter 5, and Part 2 is devoted to a detailed discussion of Chinese herbal formula strategies, methods and examples.

In late Imperial China, some physicians recorded the use of a so-called 'talking cure' in some of their cases. The technique reinterpreted an old therapeutic principle, 'announcing causes' (祝由 *zhù yóu*), and incorporated a kind of emotional counter-therapy whereby one emotional state could be counteracted by another. Emotional counter-therapy is an application of the *Inner Canon*'s five phases (五行 *wǔ xíng*).[45] For example, the fire phase is associated with the heart, and the heart with joy; the heart lodges the *shén*, and the heart-*shén* is damaged by excess joy and euphoria. According to the model's 'mutual conquest' dynamic, fear overcomes excess joy. Because fear is associated with the kidney and the water phase, and water overcomes fire, the disordered *qì* movements and relationships caused by excess joy are counteracted by fear. The following two stories illustrate the idea of an early therapeutic approach based on 'talking' and emotional manipulation.

The *Annals of the Three Kingdoms*[46] (3rd century CE) records that Huá Tuó[47] (140–208 CE) was asked to treat the governor. Huá Tuó asked for a lot of money without offering any treatment and left a letter in which he scolded the governor. The governor flew into a rage and ordered his attendants to chase and kill Huá Tuó. Because Huá Tuó had previously explained to the governor's son that the governor would be cured once he became angry, the son protected Huá Tuó. Meanwhile, the governor's rage had caused him to vomit a large amount of black blood, after which he recovered.

Ming and Qing dynasty medical works recorded Zhāng Cóngzhèng's[48] (1156–1228) skill in the technique of emotional catharsis therapy. Zhāng Cóngzhèng suggested that, where applicable, a doctor might play tricks on his patients. He felt that if the doctor's use of deceit and trickery was cunning and unpredictable, they could distract the patient's attention and change their way of looking at things. In his own *Confucians' Duties to Their Parents*,[49] Zhāng records some of his patient cases as well as some earlier reported cases. In one well-known story, a Lord with severe and constant diarrhea sent for Dr. Yáng in Shandong Province. On entering the Lord's home, Yáng did not examine or even speak with his patient. Instead, the doctor entertained his host's entire family with stories about astronomy, extreme weather and the celestial circles. Yáng's tales were

---

45 The five phases (五行) are a conceptual model that is as ancient as *yīn* and *yáng*. The five phases or elements are wood, fire, earth, metal and water. They represent five essential *qì* qualities, their relationships and transformations, that apply to all phenomena in the universe including human life

46 《三国志》 *Sān guó zhì*

47 华佗 Huá Tuó

48 张从正 Zhāng Cóngzhèng

49 《儒门事亲》 *Rú mén shì qīn*

so riveting that the Lord was engrossed and so distracted from his illness that he forgot to go to the toilet throughout the reception.

In this story, Dr. Yáng later explained to the Lord why he had administered such a treatment: 'The approach to curing this type of diarrhea is to distract the patient from their condition by asking about their hobbies and interests. Discuss Go and Chess with those who enjoy board games, discuss flutes and organs with those who enjoy music, and hold the conversation for as long as possible.' Yáng had simply talked about what his patient loved in order to distract the man's attention from his illness. As the *Inner Canon* states, treatments will not fail so long as the doctor understands what their patients loathe and adore (Qu and Garvey 2016).

Zhāng Cóngzhèng's approach to the 'talking cure' adapted the ancient ritual practice of 'announcing causes.' Wú Jūtōng[50] (c. 1758– 1836) also believed that it was necessary to announce causes whenever a doctor treats 'inner injury' (内伤 *nèi shāng*), that is, emotionally induced disorders. Wú argued that the doctor must observe their patients' mental and emotional states and search for hidden feelings such as unfulfilled wishes, frustration, accumulated thoughts or unhappiness at heart. Once they determine the root of their patient's illness, the doctor should make this known to them (Chen 2014).

Chinese medicine's so-called 'talking cures' were very different from modern psychotherapy in that the emphasis was not on patient narratives. Wú Jūtōng, for example, stressed the importance of the doctor's role in assisting patients to change their view of themselves. The doctor should dispel perplexity through spoken guidance, and transform emotions so that the patient's mental and emotional activities and responses may flourish. However, and despite its success in some recorded clinical encounters, emotional therapy and talking cures remained far less common than medicinal therapies.

Wáng Kěntáng regarded emotion-related illnesses as *qì* disorders, and favoured medicinal prescriptions for their treatment. Even Zhāng Cóngzhèng himself cautioned that emotional therapy strategies and the application of 'five phase mutual conquest' were not suitable for all patients (Chiang 2014). Thus, in general, Chinese doctors tended to use medicinal prescriptions in their treatment of mental and emotional disorders. This remains true in practice in China today.

---

50 吴鞠通 Wú Jūtōng

Today, Chinese medicine still observes the patient's lived experience and their body/person as integrated process-systems that depend on orderly *qì* movement, the harmonious interaction of *qì* and blood, and the dynamic balance of *yīn* and *yáng*. Chinese medicine diagnosis identifies disruptions on that level, and its therapeutic methods are designed to restore orderly *qì* movements and interactions. By adjusting the patient's *qì* and blood, Chinese medicine treatments create optimum circumstances whereby the *shén* and body form are unified, the three treasures (*jīng qì shén*) are strong and well integrated, the five-phase relationships are orderly, and human life unfolds.

The Inner Canon

The *Inner Canon* has a great deal to say about human life and psychological disorder, and we draw on relevant sections from many parts of the *Elementary Questions* and *Divine Pivot* throughout Part 1. Two treatises are especially helpful to understand early Chinese psychological thought. One is the *Elementary Questions* Treatise 8, 'The Secret Treatise of the Royal Library'[51] and the other is the *Divine Pivot* Treatise 8, 'Root *Shén*.'[52]

The *Inner Canon* often describes human health and illness as states of socio-political order and disorder. The *Elementary Questions* Treatise 8 sets out the famous analogy in which the responsibilities and associations of the '*yīn* and *yáng* visceral systems' (藏府 *zàng fǔ*) are described in terms of a nation, its emperor, officials, offices and transport systems.

The *Inner Canon* uses the term 神 *shén* in two distinct ways. The overall *shén* is a general concept for all aspects of human life and conscious awareness. In some respects, the *Elementary Questions* Treatise 8 identifies this role in its description of the heart-*shén* as emperor of the nation/person because as emperor it is the overall ruler.

---

51 《素问·灵兰秘典论篇》 *Sù wèn, Líng lán mì diǎn lùn piān*
52 《灵枢·本神》 *Líng shū, Běn shén*

But the heart-*shén* is also just one of the 'five *zàng shén*.'[53] A systematic account of the five *shén* is given in the *Divine Pivot*, Treatise 8.

The Elementary Questions, Treatise 8

The treatise compares a person to a nation with its governing bureaucracy of officials that coordinate and manage its *qì* resources, functions and movements. The internal visceral systems (藏府 *zàng fǔ*) are administrative officials governing orderly life activities. When describing the heart's directing influence on our life, health and body form, Treatise 8 emphasizes the importance for the ruler governing the nation to cultivate '*shén* clarity and brightness' (神明 *shén míng*). The cultivation of *shén míng* means the development of rational mentality.

Treatise 8 says the heart is the 'sovereign ruler and host' (君主 *jūn zhǔ*), whose role is to enlighten the *shén* towards brightness:

> The heart is the official functioning as ruler. *Shén*-spirit/mind brightness originates in it. …if the ruler is enlightened, his subjects are peaceful and safe… If the ruler is not enlightened, then the twelve officials are in danger.[54]

The character for 明 *míng* consists of the sun 日 *rì*, and moon 月 *yuè*: it means 'bright, radiant and clear.' *Shén* brightness is an expression for psychological development and the power and clarity of human conscious awareness. *Shén míng* refers to clear, acute senses and to a person with rational and clear insight. As ruler and host for the *shén*, the heart is responsible for cultivating *shén* brightness. Orderly, clear and bright heart-*shén* functions have positive ramifications for our person, our *qì* influences and substances, our body structures and physical appearance, and our mental and emotional life. Everyone's heart *shén* develops from a young infant's immaturity and bewilderment towards the rational maturity of the adult state. The Chinese expression, 'brighten your heart-mind to reveal your true nature'[55] describes the cultivated state. In this saying, 明心 *míng xīn* means 明神 *míng shén*

---

53 五藏神 *wǔ zàng shén* (In the *Inner Canon*, 藏 is the original character for the *zàng-yin* visceral systems. The modern simple 脏 and complex 臟 characters include the flesh radical, which denotes their physical properties. All forms of the character mean, 'the viscera that store.' We use 藏 to emphasize the 藏神 *zàng shén* properties under discussion in this book.)

54 心为君主之官，神明出焉 … … 主明则下安，主不明则十二官危。 *Xīn wèi jūn zhǔ zhī guān. Shén míng chū yān… Zhǔ míng zé xià ān. Zhǔ bù míng zé shí'èr guān wēi*

55 明心见性 '*míng xīn jiàn xìng*'

'clarity and enlightenment': the radiance of the *shén* reveals our inner nature and natural qualities.

In fact, all the *yīn* visceral systems (藏 *zàng*) contribute to psychological health and intelligence. The *Elementary Questions* Treatise 8 description of the *zàng fǔ* officials complements the *Divine Pivot* Treatise 8 discussion of their psychological resources and functions. For example, the *Elementary Questions* says that skill comes from the kidney *zàng* and in Chinese medicine the idea encompasses both physical and mental skill. In the *Divine Pivot*, the kidney stores the 志 *zhì*, the mind/memory. The kidney-*zhì*'s power and determination concentrate the mind and the *jīng*-essence. This means that any skilled achievements, whether those of a pianist, gymnast or doctor, reflect the strength and power of their kidney-*zhì* and *jīng*-essence.

The Divine Pivot, Treatise 8

In Chinese medicine, the source of life is like the root (本 *běn*) of a tree, and the title of the *Divine Pivot* Treatise 8 is the 'Root [of the] *shén*' (本神 *Běn shén*). Its title refers to the source of sentient human life, and the treatise presents each of the five *zàng* in terms of their mental and emotional responsibilities and relationships. Its discussion reflects the descriptions of their administrative responsibilities presented in the *Elementary Questions* Treatise 8.

In the *Divine Pivot* Treatise 8, Lines 21 to 30 are especially interesting for Chinese medicine psychology and cognition development (see our translation below). They describe mental faculties and staged thinking processes, which are defined in relation to one another and imply a progression of cognitive facility and relationship. And they begin with the origin of life. Lines 21 and 22 describe conception, when the female and male *jīng*-essences combine to form new life:

(21) The substance of life is called essence (精 *jīng*).

(22) Interaction of the two essences is called *shén*-spirit/mind (神).

(23) That which comes and goes with the [heart-] *shén* is called the soul (魂 *hún*).

(24) That which follows the essence exiting and entering is called the *pò* (魄).

(25) What responds to the [internal and external] environment is the heart (心 *xīn*).

(26) What the heart[-*shén*] brings out is called consciousness/ideation (意 *yì*).

(27) What consciousness/ideation stores is called memory (志 *zhì*).

(28) Because of the mind and memory, knowledge is reorganized. This is called thinking and reflection (思 *sī*).

(29) Because of thinking and reflection, one thinks for the future. This is called planning and strategy (虑 *lǜ*).

(30) Because of planning, strategy and thoughtful consideration, one makes decisions and takes actions. This is called wisdom (智 *zhì*).[56]

At conception, the ovum and sperm are the original *yīn* and *yáng jīng*-essences, and their interaction creates new life: the *shén*. The foetus' inherited *jīng-shén* provides the basic resources, information and instinctual functions needed for early life in the womb and later developmental life stages. Lines 21 and 22 state that life activities are based on the *jīng*-essence, and from there the Treatise introduces the five *zàng shén*, each of which are responsible for particular aspects of human mentality. Although the 魂 *hún* and 魄 *pò* are often translated as the '*yáng* soul' and '*yīn* soul,' this is not accurate. According to the *Book of Changes*, 'the *shén* cannot be measured by *yīn* and *yáng*,'[57] and for that reason, we prefer to use the pinyin for them.

We perceive and respond to the external world every waking moment via a constant stream of sensory information, and according to Line 25, all external matters and perceptions are received and coordinated by the heart-*shén*. The 意 *yì*-ideation is like the first phase of thinking when an idea arises in our conscious mind. Translations for 意 *yì* include 'attention,' 'intent' and 'consciousness,' so when the heart-*shén* applies itself to reception and analysis, this is the *yì*'s focus and attention. In Line 27, when the 志 *zhì*-mind takes charge of the

---

56 (21) 生之来谓之精，*Shēng zhī lái wèi zhī jīng*
   (22) 两精相搏谓之神。*Liǎng jīng xiāng bó wèi zhī shén*
   (23) 随神往来谓之魂，*Suí shén wǎi lái wèi zhī hún*
   (24) 并精出入谓之魄，*Bìng jīng chū rù wèi zhī pò*
   (25) 所以任物者谓之心。*Suǒ yǐ rèn wù zhě wèi zhī xīn*
   (26) 心有所忆谓之意，*Xīn yǐn sun yì wèi zhī yì*
   (27) 意之所存谓之志，*Yì zhī su cún wèi zhī zhì*
   (28) 因志而存变谓之思，*Yīn zhì ér cún biàn wèi zhī sī,*
   (29) 因思而远谋谓之虑，*Yīn sī ér yuan móu wèi zhī lǐ*
   (30) 因虑而处物为智。*Yīn lǐ ér chr wù wèi zhī zhì*
57 阴阳不测谓之神。*Yīn yáng bù cè wèi zhī shén*

results of perception, there is a shift towards more processual depth and complexity. *Yì*-ideation manages the recollection of images and ideas while the *zhì*-mind functions bring skillful direction and determination to our powers of concentration, memory and ambition.

The heart-*shén* receives and coordinates our perceptions and responses. Together, the *shén*-spirit/mind and *yì*-ideation perform the initial processing of sensory information to accomplish first-stage analysis and assessment. The *zhì*-mind/memory is responsible for deeper conclusions and the more refined results of cognitive and affective processing. The *shén* is stored in the heart, the *yì* in the spleen, and the *zhì* in the kidney *zàng*, and the symmetry of content in the *Elementary Questions* and *Divine Pivot* supports their connections. The spleen *zàng*'s 'transporting and transforming' (运化 *yùn huà*) of nutrient foods and liquids is the first stage of digestion. The kidney *zàng*'s second stage '*qì* transformations' (气化 *qì huà*) manage, store and protect the pure *qì* substances (the 精 *jīng*-essence) derived from digestion.

Treatise 8 describes how prolonged and excess mental and emotional states harm the *zàng* visceral systems and their *qì* influences. It names the manifestations of *zàng shén* disruption; for example, forgetfulness, confusion, misunderstanding, inability to concentrate, failure to recognize people. It draws on the differentiated *zàng shén* responsibilities and relationships to convey a sense of mental and emotional disorder and disintegration—the *hún* and *pò* fly upward, or they are scattered; the *zhì* and *yì* are confused, or disordered; the *jīng*, *shén*, *hún* and *pò* are scattered and not harmonized (Chiu 1986).

✳ ✳ ✳

Although early Chinese medicine did not develop a distinct branch of psychological medicine, it most certainly did analyze the physical, mental and emotional features, attributes and phenomena of life. Historically, Chinese medicine does not radically differentiate between the body and mind, and yet it would be wrong to assume that it sees them as one and the same. In fact, Chinese texts discuss their distinct functional activities even though the body and mind are not considered as fundamentally different in nature (Kohn 1992). These early onto-epistemics make Chinese medicine uniquely equipped to analyze and treat 'somato-psychic illnesses.'[58]

---

58 身心疾病 *shēn xīn jí bìng*

The *Inner Canon* describes the origin of human life and its postnatal mental and emotional resources and functions. According to Chinese culture and medicine, life emerges through the interaction of heaven and earth, *yáng* and *yīn*. Our prenatal resources are embodied postnatally by the three treasures, *jīng qì shén*, and the fully differentiated configurations of postnatal human life manifest in accordance with five-phase associations. Prenatal *jīng* and *shén* form the basis of postnatal life. They produce the body form, the body is the house of the *shén*, and *shén* governs the body and its external appearance.

When the body form and *shén* are unified, the five *zàng shén* function harmoniously. Orderly, integrated five *shén* activities receive and analyze sensory information and create human conscious awareness, intelligence and cognitive ability. We can observe this orderly state through the activities of their visceral systems, senses, body tissues, *qì* substances and influences. Chinese medicine's analysis of the *shén* pays particular attention to signs of disruption and disintegration occurring in any of these relationships. The five *zàng* and their administrative responsibilities, their *wǔ shén* functions, the roles of their *qì*, blood and *jīng*-essences, and their relationships to the body form and its structures are the basis of early Chinese psychological thinking and of clinical TCM psychology today.

The heart (心 *xīn*) is seen as a physical organ as well as the abode of the 神 *shén*-spirit/mind. As head of state, the heart-*shén* receives and coordinates sensory perceptions and cognitive processes, and manages our emotional responses. The translation of 心 *xīn* as 'heart-mind' highlights the Chinese convergence of structure and mentality in a single word. Correctly understood, terms like 心 *xīn* are a semantic hinge between the physical, mental and emotional resources of human life, and this explains how our physiological and mental states can be observed through external manifestations such as our complexion, demeanor, eyes and speech.

In Chinese medicine today, the overall 神 *shén* refers broadly to human life. The heart-*shén* is aligned with the resources and activities of human mentality, and with our mental and emotional disposition and behaviors. It governs our intelligence and conscious awareness. Understanding the *shén* therefore is a necessary step towards investigating the principles of TCM psychology and their basis in ancient and pre-modern Chinese psychological thinking.

Chapter 2

Human Life

The Chinese believe that each of us plays a part in the long river of human evolution. Regarding the transmission of life, early thinkers described our person as the inherited body of our parents, and in the *Mò Zǐ*[59] (*c.* 400 BCE) this is defined as 'a share of the whole.' Similarly, the *Mèng Zǐ*[60] (*c.* 300 BCE) states that 'the myriad things are fully here in me,' and 'one who knows his nature knows heaven [天]' (Ames 1993).

The Chinese see all natural phenomena, including human life, as arising spontaneously from the benevolence of the natural world (天 *tiān* 'heaven'). Consequently, the natural world is within the nature (性 *xìng*) of every human life, its unlearned biological functions and capabilities, and its *shén* qualities, character and behaviors. In this chapter, we examine the basis and origin of human life, its union with nature and the expression of *shén* in this life.

The basis of human life

The ancient Chinese believed there were two main kinds of life. The life source of sentient beings was rooted inside and tied to heaven, whereas the source of other forms of life was rooted outside and tied to earth. Three related concepts—the inner root, *shén* dynamic and *qì* set-up—speak to this idea and are part of the *Inner Canon*'s 'five circuits

---

59 墨子 Mò Zǐ (470–391 BCE), 'Master Mo,' philosopher of the Early Warring States period, founder of school of Mohism and author of the *Mò Zǐ*

60 孟子 Mèng Zǐ (372–289 BCE), 'Master Meng,' 'Mencius,' Confucian philosopher and sage

and six *qì* theory.'[61] In the *Elementary Questions*, Treatise 70 ('Great Treatise on the Five Regular Orders') it says:

> When embryos are not formed and do not develop, and if treating these cases does not result in success, this is a regular feature of the *qì*. This is the so-called 'inner root' (中根 *zhōng gēn*).
>
> Those rooted in the exterior, they too are five. Hence, the differences in generation and transformation follow the five *qì*, five colours, five categories, and five correspondences.[62]

In living creatures, the origin of life is the 'generative *qì*' (生气 *shēng qì*). Their 'inner root' (中根 *zhōng gēn*) is this generative *qì*, which is stored in the five *zàng* and emerges from within the body. Yet, life depends on more than that. According to the *Inner Canon*, the *qì* of living beings and all phenomena are vulnerable to climatic conditions and changes and must follow the five circuits and six *qì*. So, when the text notes that life and its continuation is a 'regular feature of the *qì*,' 'the *qì*' here means both the internal physiological (*shén*) *qì* and the external (environmental) *qì*. The external *qì* are the six *qì*, the climatic phenomena of wind, cold, summerheat, dampness, dryness and fire.

Treatise 70 continues:

> The one rooted inside is called '*shén* dynamic' (神机 *shén jī*). When the *shén* is gone, the dynamic stops. The one rooted outside is called '*qì* set-up' (气立 *qì lì*). When the *qì* stops circulating, generation and transformation are interrupted.[63]

Treatise 70 states that the one rooted inside is the *shén* and its life dynamic. The *shén* triggers all movement and resting so when the *shén* leaves, the dynamic follows it, vitality ceases and life ends. The *shén* and its dynamic, the *shén jī*, decides life and death.

---

61 五运六气学说 *wǔ yùn liù qì xué yuè*

62 《素问·五常政大论》：故有胎孕不育，治之不全，此气之常也。所谓中根也，根于外者亦五，故生化有别，有五气，五味，五色，五类，五宜也。
Sù wèn, Wǔ cháng zhèng dà lùn: 'Gù yǒu tāi yùn bù yù, zhì zhī bù quán, cǐ qì zhī cháng yě. Suǒ wèi zhōng gēn yě, gēn yú wài zhě yì wǔ, gù sheng huà yǒu bié, Yǒu wǔ qì, wǔ wèi, wǔ sè, wǔ lèi, wǔ yí yě'

63 《素问·五常政大论》：根于中者，命曰神机，神去则机息；根于外者，命曰气立，气止则化绝。
Sù wèn, Wǔ cháng zhèng dà lùn: 'Gēn yú zhōng zhě, mìng yuē shén jī, shén qù zé jī xi; gēn yú wài zhě, mìng yuē qì lì, qì zhǐ zé huà jué'

The generation, growth, transformation and completion of things rooted outside depend on external *qì* for their existence. This applies to plant life and other natural phenomena. They are 'rooted in the exterior' because the basis of their generative *qì* is external. They take *qì* from the outside to complete their organizational arrangements. When the *Inner Canon* speaks of the '*qì* establishment' or '*qì* set-up' (气立 *qì lì*), 气 *qì* here means the external seasons and climates, as well as the internal life functions of living creatures, and立 *lì* means the customary stages and well-known changes of *qì*. Plants only require the earth and environmental *qì* to ascend and descend to come to life, grow, transform, and be harvested and stored. For things rooted in the exterior, the basis of their generative *qì* is cut off when external *qì* influences are removed.

This external *qì*, the five circuits and six *qì*, actually applies to all things. As Treatise 70 goes on to say:

> Hence, all things have something by which they are restrained, dominated, generated, and brought to completion. Therefore, it is said that those who do not know what the circuit of a year (岁运 *suì yùn*) contributes, or whether [the arrival of] the six *qì* are similar or different, are unable to understand the processes of generation and transformation (生化 *shēng huà*). This is what it refers to.

When the *qì* of external transformations ceases, then all transformations are interrupted. All life—human, animal and plant life, germination, growth and so on—depend on the established and regular changes of *qì*, the 气立 *qì lì*. The *Inner Canon* affirms that whether rooted in their own inner core or in the exterior, 'All things have something by which they are restrained, dominated, generated and brought to completion.' This means that all natural phenomena correspond to the five phases (五行 *wǔ xíng*) and their processes of generation and transformation.

The difference with sentient creatures is that their life *qì* has its origin within the body and the *shén* is responsible for their movement and rest. The *Elementary Questions* Treatise 68 links the *shén* dynamic to the movement and rest of living beings and to the idea of entering and exiting:

> When exiting and entering ceases, the transforming activity of the *shén* dynamic vanishes. When ascending and descending stop, then the *qì* set-up is solitary and in danger.

'Exiting and entering' refers to breathing (and the energy exchange of all living beings), an essential manifestation of the *shén jī*. 'Ascending and descending' refers to the increasing and decreasing of *yīn* and *yáng*, such as the coming and going of winter-cold and summer-heat. *Yīn* and *yáng* increasing and decreasing brings about the movement and transformation of the five *qì*: generation, growth, transformation, gathering and storage. Without them, birth, growth, adulthood, aging and death cannot take place. The form and structure of all physical things and all living beings is shaped by the transformations of *qì*: this is known as *qì lì*.

The *Elementary Questions*' five circuits and six *qì* theory describes the dynamic changes of nature in detail. The *zhōng gēn*, *shén jī* and *qì lì* concepts in particular explain the associations between the changes of nature and the dynamics of life.

中根 *Inner root*

The 'central' or 'inner root' (中根 *zhōng gēn*) refers to the foundation that generates *qì* in all phenomena. The word 中 *zhōng* means 'center and core,' and 根 *gēn* means a thing's 'makeup and essential nature.' It is similar to the idea of a thing's natural disposition. In living beings, it refers to the foundation and nature of life. As the *Elementary Questions* says, 'The one rooted inside is called *shén jī* (神机)... The one rooted outside is called *qì lì* (气立).' This indicates that when the foundation of life is rooted inside, the inner root comes from the *shén* dynamic, and determines the nature of the species. For example, chicken eggs hatch chickens, while crocodile eggs hatch crocodiles. The one rooted outside comes from the cycles, changes and transformations of the seasons and climate. So while the hatching of all eggs is influenced by climatic changes and temperature, the type of hatchlings is decided by their inner root nature.

When a thing's inner root is external, its *qì* transformations are decided by the established set-up of the external *qì*, the *qì* of heaven and earth. Its inner root conforms to the correspondences and relationships of the natural world. These correspondences are described by the generation, growth, transformation, gathering and storage *qì* movements of the five phases and five circuits. The correspondences and inter-relatedness between nature and life also apply to the one rooted inside; however, its inner root is dominated by the *shén* dynamic and is concealed rather than apparent.

神机 *Shén dynamic*

神 *Shén* signifies sentient life and is the fundamental difference between sentient creatures and their natural environment. The ancients viewed the living body as comprising innumerable life mechanisms or dynamics, which together were known as the '*shén* dynamic' (神机 *shén jī*). Therefore, the *Inner Canon* states that, 'The one rooted inside is called *shén jī*. When the *shén* is gone, the dynamic ceases.' In living beings, the *shén* is the ruler of the generative life *qì* and consciousness, and the *shén* dynamic rules the processes of life and its transformations.

机 *Jī* was an ancient word for a crossbow's firing mechanism. The *Inner Canon* and later texts use this image of a trigger, this small, simple mechanism and action, to represent the idea of incipience and impetus. In the medical context, *jī* means the incipient functional mechanisms and stimulus for the generation, manifestations and complexity of life. *Shén* is the precursor of *jī* and the dominant partner determining vitality, and therefore, 'Once the *shén* is gone, the mechanism stops.'

According to Wáng Bīng,[64] the *shén* dynamic is the unfathomable changes and transformations of *yīn* and *yáng*. It is the essence of life, the sum of all the incipient *qì* generation dynamics that occur within living organisms. It utilizes external physical environmental conditions to set up the '*qì* mechanism' (气机 *qì jī*) producing life activities. In Chinese medicine the *qì* mechanism is the self-regulating, self-organizing ascending/descending and inward/outward movements of *qì*. The *qì jī* maintains homeostasis, unity and physiological viability, and supports the facility to utilize external environmental conditions relatively independently. The external conditions themselves are established through the *qì* set-up (气立 *qì lì*).

The *shén* dynamic determines the generative and transforming processes producing life, and it coordinates the balance and unity between the living body and its external environment. Three points are important for understanding this idea. First, the *shén jī* (神机) determines life and death: the presence of the *shén* provokes the

---

64 王冰 Wáng Bīng (*c.* 710–805 CE) edited the *Inner Canon* in 762 and is one of its most famous commentators

life *qì* dynamic (气机) and this is the inner root of all sentient life events. Preparing the foetus for birth, for example, and the occasion of pregnancy itself, are determined by the *shén jī*. In fact, all life processes unfold from the interior, are revealed externally, and are controlled and oriented by the *shén jī*.

Second, the *shén jī* determines the trend of pathological changes, and prognosis is related to the vitality or dysfunction of the *shén jī*. The *Elementary Questions* Treatise 14 says: 'When essence *qì* fades, the *ying*-nutrient and *wei*-defense *qì* vanish, and when the *shén* leaves the disease does not heal.' In the clinical setting, we see some patients with severe diseases recover quickly, while some with mild illnesses are slow to recover. *Shén jī* plays an important and sometimes decisive role in the susceptibility to, process of, and recovery from disease.

Third, the *shén jī*'s life processes are similar to metabolism. The *shén jī* concept and the science of physiology are both concerned with how living beings are continuously undergoing processes of construction and destruction, anabolism and catabolism, assimilation and excretion, increasing and decreasing. These life processes are the *qì* transformations of the *shén jī*. They are Wáng Bīng's 'unfathomable changes and transformations of *yīn* and *yáng*.'

Living beings are constantly exchanging material and energy with their environment—the intake of food, water and air through digestion and respiration, the transformations producing essence *qì*, the excretion of waste and generation of new materials. Assimilation and excretion, the processes absorbing and discharging materials and energy to the environment, confirm and define the relationship between living creatures and the natural world. These belong to the processes of *qì lì*, and in this way, the *qì* set-up also shares some similarities with metabolic theory.

The living human body obtains *qì* from the natural environment through the established processes of *qì lì*. The *shén* dynamic acts on the intake of environmental *qì* influences, transforming them into essential substances, such as nutritive and defense *qì*, blood and fluids, through *zàng fǔ qì* transformations. In this way, the body is constructed. Meanwhile, the wastes produced from *qì* transformations are expelled through the established processes of the *qì* set-up, the *qì lì*.

气立 Qi set-up

The word 气 qì has many meanings and encompasses all processes of generation and transformation. In terms of the natural environment, it refers to climatic conditions, rhythms and cycles; and in terms of human life, it refers to physiological functions, movements and transformations. The word 立 lì means to root, set up and establish.

The *Inner Canon* calls the external conditions and qì activities that support life, the 'qì set-up' (气立 qì lì). Its meaning has two parts. One concerns the natural environment and external conditions. Living organisms must acquire and conform to these established qì transformations and changes. The other concerns the regulation of absorption and excretion that maintains the balance between the internal and external environments. In sentient beings this occurs through the *shén jī* entering and exiting, the breath.

If something does not belong to the five categories of living creatures (hairy, feathered, naked, scaly or armored), then the generative qì depends on external things to be established. All living creatures rely on the qì set-up of their environmental conditions to align their vital functions with the ascending and descending, inward and outward qì dynamics of the natural world. In living creatures, the qì lì is this association between their external environment and internal life activities. That is why, when these external influences are removed, the generative qì is cut off: 'The one rooted outside is called qì lì. If the qì stops circulating, generation and transformation are interrupted.'

The externally established qì lì is the summation of all qì dynamics. It is the established and self-organizing processes of qì transformations that are an extension of the 'movement of nature' (天运 tiān yùn). They are bound to five-phase (五行 wǔ xíng) natural law and its 'cycles of engendering and restraining.'[65] They are bound to the 'five circuits' (五运 wǔ yùn) and 'six qì' (六气 liù qì), and the established qì transformations producing all phenomena. To understand these qì processes of generation, growth, transformation, gathering and storage, the *Inner Canon* says we must know the 'circuit of the year' (岁运 suì yùn) and the arrival of the six qì. It says that the generation and transformation of all things and all living creatures can be distinguished according to the five qì, five flavors, five colors, five categories and five correspondences.

---

65 相生相克 xiāng shēng xiāng kè

Therefore, *qì lì* is bi-directional. The one rooted inside originates from *shén jī* and its vitality is concealed. The one rooted outside responds to the generating, transporting, engendering and restraining *qì* processes that establish life. To establish the *shén jī* rooted inside, life must respond to the external *qì* and accomplish the generation and transformation processes of the *qì lì*.

The origin of human life

The Chinese consider human life a part of nature, and life vitality a part of the power of nature. We find the same notion in the early medical texts. For example, the title of the *Elementary Questions* Treatise 3, 'On How the Generative *Qì* Communicates with Heaven/Nature,'[66] means the life *qì* of all beings is an expression of the natural order. In *Explaining and Analyzing Characters* (121 CE), 神 *shén* is glossed: 'nature creates the myriad things.'[67] In the Han dynasty dictionary, 天神 *tiān shén* is the 'power of nature'—it exists everywhere, creating and driving everything in the universe. While here we translate 天神 *tiān shén* as the sovereign, mysterious and unpredictable 'power of nature,' Thomas Cleary (1981) and Richard Wilhelm (1984) use 'celestial mind,' and 'heavenly consciousness,' respectively for their English translations of *The Secret of the Golden Flower*.[68] The *Golden Flower* is a Chinese self-cultivation text, with practices that are thought to go back to an 8th-century Buddhist–Daoist current connected to the famous adept Lǚ Dòngbīn.[69]

Although the 'power of nature' (天神 *tiān shén*) is immaterial and invisible, in Chinese culture it creates and drives everything in the universe. Different countries and religions have recognized a supreme and dominating force and given it different names, such as God and Allah. Chinese philosophical currents also recognized a special controlling power in cosmic space. In fact, in Chinese language, a close synonym for 天神 *tiān shén* is 天德 *tiān dé*, which means a benevolent 'god.' Both terms encompass the notion of heavenly kindness and benevolence. On its own, 天 *tiān* means 'sky' and 'the heavens' above human beings, and infers the existence of a dominating force.

---

66 《素问 · 生气通天论》 *Sù wèn, Shēng qì tōng tiān lùn*
67 《说文解字》： **天神**引出万物者也。 *Shuō wén jiě zì:* '***Tiān shén** yǐn chū wàn wù zhě yě*'
68 《太乙金華宗旨》 *Tài yǐ jīn huá zōng zhǐ* (first published around 1680)
69 呂洞賓 Lǚ Dòngbīn (b. 796)

The power of nature (天神 *tiān shén*) is considered the force behind the eternal dynamic of the universe.

天神 *The power of nature*

In ancient times, 天 *tiān* referred to a higher ancestor, and then to the ancestors' dwelling place. Then, as a more nature-based worldview replaced magical and ancestor explanations (from the end of the Warring States period), the meaning of 天 *tiān* reflected that change. Though often translated as 'heaven,' its meaning is actually more like 'nature,' such as in the *Mèng Zǐ* (*c.* 300 BCE), where heaven/nature (天) was the source of human nature and mentality: 'To the mind pertains the role of thinking... This is what heaven has given to me' (Unschuld 2009; Zhang 2002).

Wilhelm (1984) explains that early Confucian and Daoist thinkers saw *tiān shén* as the center of emptiness, and Cleary's translation (1981) calls it 'unconditioned consciousness.' But he begins by simply stating its naturalness: 'Naturalness is called the Way [Dào, cosmic law].' These explanations draw our attention to another important idea that is characteristic of the early Chinese worldview: 'spontaneity' (自然 *zì rán*). In the *Classic of the Law and Its Power*,[70] for example, 自然 *zì rán*'s original meaning, 'what is so of itself,' expressed the idea of an inclusive, self-generating, all-enfolding harmony. Its meaning has broadened over the centuries so that today both *zì rán* and *tiān shén* are often translated as 'nature.'

The notion of spontaneous self-generation (自然 *zì rán*) indicates that all phenomena are both self-determinate and determined by all other phenomena. Related to this perspective is 'the continuity of being,' and the interconnectedness of all things. This is why the *Classic of the Law and Its Power* advocates the law of non-action (无为 *wú wéi*) and spontaneity (自然 *zì rán*) (Lai 2006). Just as Daoism considers life a perceptible form of the *dào* (道 cosmic law), Chinese culture sees all living creatures as arising from the power of nature. The spontaneous unfolding of the universe is organized through principle (理 *lǐ*) and share or allotment (分 *fēn*). The heavenly power of *lǐ*-principle manifests in us as our life-destiny (命 *mìng*); the heavenly destiny of specific individual *fēn*-allotments manifests as each person's inner nature (性 *xìng*).

---

70 《道德经》 *Dào dé jīng*

人神 *Human life*

The Chinese call human life 人神 *rén shén*, a term that infers human life is a manifestation of *tiān shén*. They say that, 'Of all living creatures the human being is divine (灵 *líng*).'[71] Because it has taken so many years of evolution to create human life, and because humans are the cleverest of all creatures, the Chinese consider human beings a special manifestation of the power of nature (see Figure 2.1).

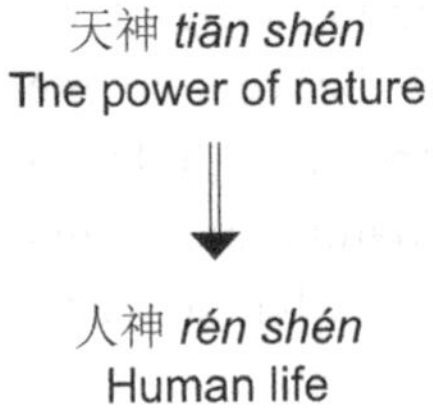

天神 *tiān shén*
The power of nature

⇓

人神 *rén shén*
Human life

Figure 2.1: The power of nature generates human life

Rén shén manifests as the appearance and movements of a human being, their way of speaking and responding, their mental and emotional behaviors and activities. Extraordinary abilities and talents such as genius and virtuosity are called 天才 *tiān cái*, meaning 'natural endowment,' so the Chinese believe that *tiān cái* are given by the power of nature rather than by one's parents. The power of nature generates human life, and the origins of human life develop through three stages: the root *shén* (本神 *běn shén*), initiating *shén* (元神 *yuán shén*) and acquired *shén* (识神 *shí shén*) (see Figure 2.2). These three aspects of *shén* are the subject of the next chapter.

---

71 人为万物之灵 *Rén wéi wàn wù zhī líng*

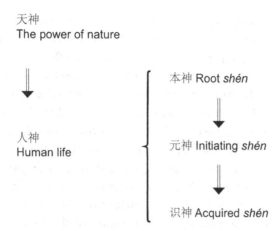

Figure 2.2: Human life, the shén, *has three aspects*

精神 *Essence shén*

The 精 *jīng*-essence and 神 *shén*-spirit/mind both feature in early discussions of the origin of life. The *Inner Canon* states that the *shén* is produced at conception when the male and female *jīng* interact. In a passage that echoes the *Divine Pivot* Treatise 8, the *Grand Basis*[72] specifically includes the body form and its relationship with *jīng*-essence and *shén*:

> When the two [male and female *jīng-shén*] conjugate, they unite to shape a physical form [形 *xíng*]. They always come into being before the body [because they provide its initial endowment of vitality as well as its form]. This is called 精 *jīng*. (Sivin 1987, p.149)

The idea behind Chinese medicine's *jīng shén* is that essence is the root of life. Postnatal essence produces sperm in men and ova in women; and for a couple to conceive, both the ovum and sperm must have the root *shén* within. Then, the interaction of the female and male *jīng*-essences (*yīn* and *yáng*) produces new life, which is regarded as the *shén*.

The parental ovum and sperm are the new individual's inherited (prenatal) 精神 *jīng shén*. The inherited *jīng* is their 'original' *yīn* and *yáng*, and the inherited *shén* is the psychological resources carried by their initiating *shén* (元神 *yuán shén*). This new configuration

---

72 《太素》 *Tài sù* (c. 656)

of inherited resources, the prenatal *jīng shén*, instigates and guides the development of the new human life in-utero. After birth, diet, respiration, education and other life experiences influence and cultivate the postnatal *jīng shén*. Thus, medically, the patient's *jīng shén* consist of before and after birth (prenatal and postnatal) influences.

Our prenatal *jīng shén* resources are embodied by the *jīng qì shén* (精气神), the 'three treasures' (三宝 *sān bǎo*). The three treasures signify prenatal life resources because from them the full energetic configurations of postnatal human life manifest according to five-phase (五行 *wǔ xíng*) correspondences and relationships. The 'five postnatal spirit/minds' (五神 *wǔ shén*) differentiate from the initiating *shén*, and their differentiation mirrors the generation of the 'five *yīn* visceral systems' (五藏 *wǔ zàng*). Together, the *jīng shén*, three treasures and 'five *zàng shén*' (五藏神 *wǔ zàng shén*) allowed the *Inner Canon* authors to describe the variety and complexity of human life, as we shall see in Chapter 4.

✳ ✳ ✳

The *Zhuāng Zǐ*'s (4th century BCE) 'one 气 *qì* through Heaven and Earth' sums up the early worldview of human life as one with nature. Chinese philosophy's *yīn/yáng* and five-phase correspondences further expound the inter-relatedness of nature and human life. *Yīn/yáng* and five-phase natural law, including the dynamics of the five circuits and six *qì*, describes the nature of our internal and external environments and ensures that the balance between them is relatively stable. The *Inner Canon*'s *zhōng gēn*, *shén jī* and *qì lì* concepts explain the connections between natural cycles and changes and the mechanisms of life.

In the *Inner Canon*, the *zhōng gēn*, *shén jī* and *qì lì* represent different components of life, the different stages of its transformation and generation. Whether the inner root is embedded internally is determined by the *shén* dynamic, while the inner root embedded externally is established by the environmental *qì* set-up. From the *Inner Canon* we find that the *qì* set-up, both the internal physiological *qì* set-up and the external climatic *qì* set-up, is bound to the theory of the five circuits and six *qì* and the generation and transformation processes of the five phases. These ideas express the unity of heaven and human life.[73]

On the one hand, the inner root encompasses the independent and coordinated roles of the *shén* dynamic and *qì* set-up. The *shén* dynamic and *qì* set-up work independently and cooperatively so that the activities of life can proceed according to natural law. On the other hand, the inner root explains their common properties: the *shén* dynamic and *qì* set-up are both responsible for maintaining the *qì* dynamic, the ascending, descending, inward and outward movements of *qì* that harmonize *yīn* and *yáng*, regulate *qì* and blood, and maintain life activities over time.

In Chinese culture, life emerges through the interaction of heaven and earth, *yáng* and *yīn*. The prenatal *jīng* and *shén* are a *yīn/yáng* pair that together form the basis of postnatal life and produce the body form. The *qì* influences of postnatal human life occur at the intersection of the *jīng* and *shén*, and when the kidney holds the *jīng*-essence, and the *shén qì* homes to the heart,[74] the *jīng shén* relationship is reflected in the postnatal *yáng*-fire and *yīn*-water relationship of the heart and kidney *zàng*. The basis for these relationships and for the transmission of life is best described by the three aspects of *shén*.

---

73 天人合一 *tiān rén hé yī*

74 神气舍心 *shén qì shě xīn* (from the *Divine Pivot*, Treatise 54). The phrase refers to the prenatal *shén*. 舍 *Shě* means 'home' and 'residence,' and the phrase describes how during gestation, the *shén qì* makes its way to, and settles in, the heart *zàng*

Chapter 3

The Three Aspects
of *Shén*

Every human life has three aspects of *shén*. The three aspects are similar to the idea of 'levels' or 'layers' of human mentality that include before birth (prenatal) and after birth (postnatal) stages of development. The three aspects provide a comprehensive explanation of the innate and acquired characteristics and abilities of human psychology. The potential interactions between a person's prenatal and postnatal aspects of *shén* have far-reaching implications for their mental, emotional, psychological and character development.

The three aspects are:

- 本神 ***Běn shén***, the root and source of the *shén*, as in the title of the *Divine Pivot* Treatise 8.[75] The root *shén* (本神) is the accumulation of experiences from all our ancestors that have been acquired and distilled by the course of human evolution. The root *shén* is the root of life. It is inherited from the parents and is the 'life force' in a hidden state before life begins.

- 元神 ***Yuán shén***, as posited by Tang dynasty Daoism and incorporated into the medical lexicon by renowned physician and author Lǐ Shízhēn,[76] is the initiating *shén*. The initiating *shén* arises at conception and instigates life. It carries the new individual's many potentials and abilities, including instinctual abilities and functions, that are derived from the root *shén*.

---

75 《灵枢·本神》 *Líng shū, Běn shén*
76 李时珍 Lǐ Shízhēn (1518–1593)

- 识神 *Shí shén*, the acquired *shén*, is derived from the initiating *shén*. The acquired *shén* comprises the activities and sensations of our conscious awareness, and is influenced by our postnatal environment. The acquired *shén* receives and responds to the stimulus and influence of family, education and environment.

Every person inherits their original, primary essence and *shén* at conception. When female and male *jīng*-essence (the ovum and sperm) combine and produce a new life, they produce the initiating *jīng* and *shén*, the prenatal 'life material' and 'life power' for basic developmental information and instinctual functions. All three aspects of the *shén*—the root and source of *shén*, the original initiating *shén* and the acquired *shén*—contribute to our personal traits, mental and emotional resources, character, personality and intelligence.

Although it frequently mentions the *shén*, the *Inner Canon* does not specifically differentiate between these three aspects or levels. In the Tang dynasty (618–907), the *Yellow Emperor's Hidden Talisman Canon*[77] alluded to the prenatal and postnatal *shén* when it stated:

> People know the *shén* of *shén*, but they do not know the no *shén* of *shén*.[78] (1999/[Unknown] *c*. 8th century)

The quote mentions *shén* 神 four times, but each has a different connotation. *The Hidden Talisman Canon* is a Daoist text associated with inner cultivation; and another source for early conceptions of the pre- and postnatal *shén* is *The Secret of the Golden Flower*,[79] also said to date from the Tang.

The Daoist meditative practices in the *Golden Flower* attempt to open the 'golden flower' of the light of the mind—an ineffable accomplishment of inner self-cultivation. The *Golden Flower* speaks of prenatal primal consciousness and postnatal knowing consciousness, using the terms 元神 *yuán shén* (the 'initiating *shén*') for the 'no *shén* of *shén*,' and 识神 *shī shén* (the 'acquired *shén*') for the '*shén* of *shén*.' The *Hidden Talisman Canon's* '*shén* of *shén*,' and the *Golden Flower's* 'acquired *shén*,' are both referring to the postnatal conscious awareness and cognitive activities of the acquired *shén* (识神 *shí shén*).

---

77 《黄帝阴符经》 *Huáng dì yīn fú jīng, c*. 8th century CE
78 '人知其神之神，而不知不神之所以神。' *'Rén zhī qí shén zhī shén, ér bù zhī bù shén zhī suǒ yǐ shén'*
79 《太乙金華宗旨》 *Tài yǐ jīn huá zōng zhǐ* (For translations in English see Cleary 1981, and Wilhelm 1984)

Because the initiating *shén* (元神) exists before birth, it was considered part of the primal *qì* that pervades the whole universe. Daoist meditators placed great importance on it as the essence of 'spiritual' consciousness. As a complex of the influences and perceptions of sensory awareness, the acquired *shén* was considered 'ordinary' consciousness. These ideas become more prominent from the late Tang and in the Song dynasties (Qu and Garvey 2009a).

The three aspects of *shén* explain how every person's *shén* incorporates prenatal and postnatal influences and resources. In premodern Chinese psychological thought, the initiating *shén* is preceded by its source, the root *shén*. The root *shén* is the source of postnatal life, the initiating *shén* is the origin of life activities, and these two are the basis of the postnatal acquired *shén*.

本神 Root *shén*

The title of the *Divine Pivot* Treatise 8 is 'The Root [of the] *Shén*' (本神 *Běn shén*). *Běn shén* means the 'source and core of human life and mentality,' our innate root *shén* influences and abilities. When *the Elementary Questions* Treatise 13 says, 'If in possession of the *shén*, life prospers, if the *shén* is lost, life perishes,'[80] the *shén* here refers to the root *shén*.

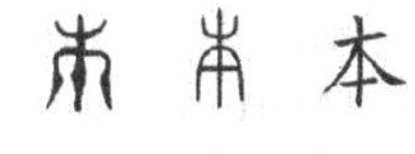

Figure 3.1: Early pictographs and modern character for 本 běn-root

The earliest form of 本 *běn* is shown on the left. Although the character has changed over time, its meaning remains the same as when it appeared in the Han dynasty dictionary *Explaining and Analyzing Characters* (121 CE). The entry says: 'Under the tree is the root.'[81] The tree grows above the earth and its root is hidden below ground, and in Chinese medicine, the source of life is like the root (本) of a tree. The etymology of the character illustrates that the root *shén* is the innate core of human life: its nature is hidden and implicit. The small horizontal line under the earth in the later two forms of

---

80 《素问·移精变气论篇》：得神者昌，失神者亡。*Sù wèn, Yí jīng biàn qì lùn piān: 'De shén zhě chāng, shī shén zhě wáng'*

81 《说文解字》：木下曰本。*Shuō wén jiě zì: 'Mù xià yuē běn'*

the character (center and right) replaces the bulging root areas shown in the pictograph on the left. These allude to the inner core of the tree's root system, its inner root (中根 *zhōng gēn*). The inner core is likened to the root *shén*, which holds the innate conditions, archetypes and instincts that are the root nature (天性 *tiān xìng*) of human mentality. All life's mysteries are kept there.

The term 'root *shén*' (本神) is synonymous with the 'source *shén*' (原神 *yuán shén*). In Chinese, we often use the expression 本源, 原本 '*běn yuán, yuán běn*' to mean the 'earliest source or origin.' The entry for 源 *yuán*-source in *Explaining and Analyzing Characters* is: 'The root of water.'[82]

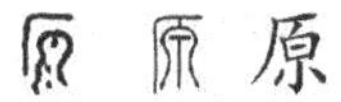

原　原　原

Figure 3.2: Early pictographs for 源 yuán-source and 原 yuán-source, and the modern character for 原 yuán-source

This is its early pictograph on the left. The inner part represents clear, pure water, and the outer part surrounding it is a mountain or cliff. The Han dynasty dictionary says: 'The underground source of spring water is the one hundred sources.'[83] The three drops in the pictograph depict water emerging from deep within the core of the mountain, and can be seen as the three treasures, the *jīng qì shén*. The second (middle) image is an early form of 原 *yuán* (on the right), which also means the 'source.' The inner part of the character represents the root, and the dictionary explains that it is the 'Root source of the source, [which] takes a very long time to accumulate.'[84] The modern simplified character (image on the right) has lost its original meanings.

The evolution of human life has also taken a very long time, and the root *shén* is the accumulated and distilled life and survival experiences and abilities of all our biological ancestors. We know that our evolutionary ancestors include our animal ancestors because humans and animals share many biological characteristics. The root *shén* also carries all the concentrated abilities acquired during human evolution, such as learning and language abilities, imagination,

---

82   《说文》：原，水本也。 *Shuō wén: 'Yuán, shuǐ běn yě'*
83   《说文》：泉水始所出为百源。 *Shuō wén: 'Quán shuǐ shǐ suǒ chū wèi bǎi yuán'*
84   《说文》：本原之原。积成非是者久矣。 *Shuō wén: 'Běn yuán zhī yuán. Jī chéng fēi shì zhě jiǔ yǐ'*

creativity, cognition, comprehension, self-awareness and intelligence. Because these abilities are partly decided by the prenatal aspects of the *shén*, in China we say that, whether a child can or cannot be educated is largely due to the root *shén*.

The distilled life abilities and survival experiences of our ancestors are stored and carried by the root *shén*. The root *shén* also carries racial, familial and individual characteristics, such as psychological characteristics and personality traits. In this way, a genetic predisposition to certain illnesses, including mental and emotional illnesses, can be considered the reappearance of characteristics that are inherent in previous generations and some ancestral archetypes. In the West, it was Carl Jung (1875–1961) who proposed the existence of universal or archetypal forms that concentrate generations of human experiences and emotions, and we return to this coincidence in Chapter 7.

Everyone experiences a different heart-*shén* road, and the Chinese believe that the collective experiences of a person's heart-*shén* road leave their mark on their individual *shén*. When extraordinary, terrible or frightening experiences make a deep impression on our inner world, they are 'engraved in the bones and imprinted on the heart.'[85] The impact of 'engraved in the bones' experiences leaves traces and effects that are stored deeply within the root *shén* and become a feature of our person, part of our psychological nature.

From ancient times, all humanity's life experiences are distilled and transferred to memories stored within the root *shén*, the source of human psychology. The kidney *zàng* governs the bones; it stores the *zhì*-mind/memory, the life essence and the root source of life. So the 'engraved in the bones' expression means that when significant experiences leave their mark on a person, this is transferred to the person's initiating *shén* and then deposited in their root *shén* (see Figure 3.5). Thus in Chinese psychological thinking, the traces and effects of our ancestors' heart roads, the life and survival experiences that deeply affected their root *shén*, became part of the survival influences and abilities that were passed on from one generation to the next. This is why dangerous or life-threatening experiences are not only acquired or learned in our own lifetime by the acquired *shén*. When 'engraved in the bones' experiences are transferred to the next generation, we may, for example, instinctively fear snakes or darkness,

---

85 刻骨铭心 *Kè gǔ míng xīn* (Chinese saying)

even though we have had no personal experience of such dangers. When we face such dangers, our instinctual fight or flight response is almost instant due to the rapid secretion of epinephrine from the adrenal glands and increased heart rate.

Related to the idea of our individual root *shén*, is the idea of ancestral and group types of root *shén*. There are country and national types of root *shén* too,[86] although the term for these is 国魂 *guó hún*, not 国神 *guó shén*. Considering the root *shén* as the depository of evolutionary, ancestral and archetypal information collected over countless generations, it is difficult to imagine, much less convey, the vast depth and complexity of our root *shén* influences.

元神 Initiating *shén*

Once the parental *jīng*-essences conceive a new life, this first, primary instance is the 'initiating spirit/mind' (元神 *yuán shén*). It is the root *shén* (本神) that generates the original or initiating *shén*-spirit/mind (元神). As the material basis of fertility, the essence of both parents must have the root *shén* to conceive life—if either the sperm or ovum do not have this, they are infertile. When carrying root *shén* life information, the inherited (parental) *jīng shén* provide the foetus with life information, developmental resources and instinctual functions. After conception, the first unfolding of these primary life influences transmits the new individual's root *shén* allotment as the foetal body begins to take form. This is the initiating *shén* that guides growth and development so, if after conception there is no initiating *shén*, the foetus will die. The foetus with initiating *shén* will develop and its life will unfold according to the natural allotment of its inherited *jīng shén*.

Basic human life functions, instincts and the timing of developmental stages are governed by the initiating *shén*. The initiating *shén* drives basic functions such as heart beat, breathing, eating and sleeping, and instigates the different stages of human growth, development and reproduction. When it is present, life continues; but without the initiating *shén*'s drive and stimulation, life ceases. An illustration of the initiating *shén* may be observed in cases of injury to the cerebral cortex that cause the patient to enter a vegetative state. In this state, initiating *shén* activities (respiration

---

86 For example, 中国精神 *zhōng guó jīng shén* ('Chinese essence *shén*'), and 华夏民族精神 *huá xià mín zú jīng shén* ('Chinese nationality essence *shén*')

and cardiac functions) persist when the acquired *shén*'s cognitive functions and conscious awareness of self and environment are absent.

The root and initiating *shén* are the prenatal aspects of *shén*. They are for the most part deeply hidden and not directly accessible to the conscious mind. During gestation, the initiating *shén* is within the developing foetus's inherited *yīn* and *yáng* essences. After birth, prenatal resources, including the root source of the *shén,* are stored in the 'lifegate' (命 门 *mìng mén*) within the kidneys. The *Golden Flower* said that the initiating *shén* resides in the square inch between and behind the eyes, and later, Lǐ Shízhēn (1518–1593) confirmed that the initiating *shén* resides in the brain.[87]

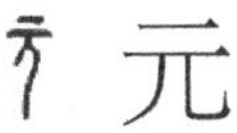

Figure 3.3: The ancient pictograph (left) and modern character (right) for 元 *yuán-initiating, original, primary*

In *Explaining and Analyzing Characters*, the entry for 元 *yuán* is, 'the beginning,'[88] meaning 'the first, primary or earliest beginning.' The character is composed of two horizontal lines (二) representing heaven and earth, and two lines underneath the earth showing the germination of a seed, the very beginning of life. The 'sprout' on the left begins to grow downward and the one on the right is just beginning to turn upward to emerge from the soil. In English, 元 *yuán* is often translated as 'origin' or 'primary.' An example of its meaning appears in the Chinese word for the Western 'New Year's Day,' 元旦 (*yuán dàn*). To the meaning of *yuán* (beginning), the word adds 旦 *dàn* (dawn), a character that shows the sun rising above the horizon.

The meanings of 原 *yuán*-source and 元 *yuán*-origin/initiating are similar, and many authors today treat them as synonymous. In Wieger (1965), 元 is 'the first cause, origin, principle,' and 原 is also the 'origin,' and 'source.' However, the 原 *yuán*-source is like 'a spring that gushes out from a hill.' 原 *Yuán* keeps to its original state and is closer to the idea of 本 *běn*-root; whereas, 元 *yuán* begins action and initiates something. Wieger's entries are based on the Han dynasty dictionary *Explaining and Analyzing Characters*.

87 '脑为元神之府'。 *'Nǎo wèi yuán shén zhī fǔ'*

88 《说文解字》：元者，始也。 *Shuō wén jiě zì: 'Yuán zhě, shǐ yě'*

In the medical context, 元 *yuán* means the 'origin' of and the power 'initiating' a human life. *Yuán*-initiating refers to the undifferentiated *qì* influences instigating and maintaining the impetus of life. Its meaning is similar to the 'one,' the 太極 *tài jí* or 'great ultimate,' the undifferentiated source of all phenomena (Zhang 2002). The *tài jí* represents the oneness before *yīn* and *yáng*, heaven and earth; it is the great ancestor of all things. The initiating *shén* too is undifferentiated life energy: it carries a new life's root *shén* allotment, a new configuration of inherited resources; it governs our unconscious and instinctive drives and mental activities. There is no cognition, memory or analysis as such during embryo stage.

In the three aspects of the *shén* model, life comes from the root (本) *shén* influences inherited from our parents and ancestors. The initiating (元) *jīng shén* contains our life resources in their primary undifferentiated state. This initiating *qì* information is the precursor and substrate of all life processes: it precedes the divisions and transformations of *yīn* and *yáng*, the development of form, substance and structure. It is through the initiating *shén* that instinctual responses and activities are passed on from one generation to the next.

The medical importance of the initiating *shén* is that it carries inherited and ancestral life information from the parental essences. A problem at the level of the initiating *shén* is transferred to the acquired *shén* and distributed to the five postnatal *shén*, their pathways and relationships, and their mental, emotional and sensory resources (see Figure 3.6). These kinds of psychological problems tend to be intractable and can be very serious.

Instincts and drives

The initiating *shén* carries the inborn instinctual abilities, behaviors and preferences that drive our postnatal physiological needs. Inherited instincts, abilities and preferences in turn are derived from the ancestral orientations of the root *shén*. For example, developmental milestones are determined by root *shén* influences, and at the proper time the initiating *shén* instigates the necessary processes and instinctual drives. Consequently, sexual drives and the ability to reproduce arise as we reach the appropriate stage of physical maturity and strength.

When the initiating *qì* fails, so does its regulation of normal, orderly physical growth, and developmental abnormalities are manifestations of this failure. For example, gigantism occurs when the timely initiating influences of kidney *qì* fail to regulate and curtail bone growth. Conversely, dwarfism will result if the initiating *qì* fails to stimulate bone growth, or slows bone growth earlier than normal.

Instinctual responses and activities such as eating and sex are necessary for human life to continue, as are our instinctive abilities to recognize and respond to danger. Generally speaking, it is the initiating *shén* that takes over in times of danger. At such times, we react instinctively: almost instantly the initiating *shén* connects with and releases unusual strength, speed or clarity, for example, or other abilities that are not normally available to us. The initiating *shén* quickly converts root *shén* experiences and abilities and transfers them to the postnatal life situation. Today we call these 'the adrenal response.' In Chinese psychological thought, the adrenal response is an example of root and initiating *shén* responses at the level of the kidney-lifegate (lodging the source 原 *yuán*) and brain (lodging the origin 元 *yuán*).

Each of us has inborn preferences, dislikes and desires. Some people prefer sweet foods, some like alcohol; some are drawn to the color red, others to blue; some fear the sea, others love the sea. According to the three aspects model, our root and initiating *shén* allotment carries and transfers particular inclinations and behaviors. To this extent, the prenatal *shén* affects our mental activities and psychological development; it influences and guides our postnatal psychological responses and actions; it shapes our personality and the quality of our relationships.

Prenatal and postnatal life

Human prenatal life lasts from conception to birth, and postnatal life begins after birth. In Chinese medicine, the expression 'before heaven' (先天 *xiān tiān*) means 'prenatal life,' and 'after heaven' (后天 *hòu tiān*) means 'postnatal life.' As the innate core of human mentality, the root *shén* is the 'prenatal [part of the] prenatal'[89] *shén*. As the beginning of a new human life, the initiating *shén* carries the root *shén* allotment and is the 'prenatal postnatal'[90] *shén*. It is the original dynamic of life. It governs innate and instinctive life functions such as breathing, digestion and heartbeat.

---

89 先天之先天 *xiān tiān zhī xiān tiān*
90 先天之后天 *xiān tiān zhī hòu tiān*

The *Canon of Difficult Issues*[91] (*c.* 100 CE) Issue 8 says that the 'source' (原 *yuán*) of life *qì* is the 'dynamic *qì*' (动气 *dòng qì*) located between the two kidneys. The 'lifegate' (命门 *mìng mén*) within the kidneys is also called the source of life because the kidney-lifegate stores our root *shén* influences and our inherited and acquired *jīng*-essences. The dynamic *qì* and lifegate are the origin of the triple burner (三焦 *sān jiāo*), which distributes the 'source *qì*' (原气 *yuán qì*) throughout the body. The original water and fire of the lifegate and the dynamic *qì* begin the movement and differentiations that produce the channel system, the five *zàng* and six *fŭ*, the body form, its structures, tissues and substances.

In postnatal life, the source *qì* is the life information that arises from the lifegate. The *sān jiāo* is the special envoy that separates the undifferentiated influences of the source *qì* and distributes them to the visceral and channel systems. The source points (原穴 *yuán xué*) on the 12 channels are where the source *qì* influences 'stop and rest.' This is why we stimulate source points to regulate and harmonize postnatal *qì* movements and transformations. After birth, the initiating *shén* resides in the brain, the root and essence of human life is kept in the lifegate within the kidneys, and the *shén qì* comes out at the heart. Together the root *shén* and initiating *shén* are the basis of our postnatal conscious awareness, and the *shén* lodging in the heart after birth oversees this third aspect of *shén*, the acquired *shén*.

Figures 3.4 and 3.5 represent the developmental stages, psychological levels, and relationships between the three aspects of *shén*. In the upper part of both diagrams:

- 识 *shì* 'knowing and understanding' is postnatal conscious awareness. The acquired *shén* perceives, analyzes and responds to life experiences. The upper part of the diagrams represents the observable activities of postnatal life, like a tree's branches and leaves.

In the middle parts:

- 元 *yuán* 'primary, origin, initiating' represents the beginning of life, conception and gestation, when our inherited life information, physical and psychological attributes, instincts and abilities, begin to take form. This is the 'prenatal postnatal' stage when the initiating *shén* achieves the in-utero transition between

---

91   《难经》 *Nán jīng*

inherited attributes and potentials and the acquired *shén* (识神). This part is like a tree's heartwood and root system.

In the lower parts of Figures 3.4 and 3.5:

- 本 *běn* 'the root and source' is the prenatal source of *shén*: it is deeply hidden, like the inner core (中根 *zhōng gēn*) of the tree's roots.

The root *shén* is the accumulation of psychological experiences that have been acquired, deposited and distilled by the course of human evolution. Even though its nature is hidden, latent and implicit, it has considerable influence on our psychological traits. It is the foundation of the initiating *shén*. The initiating *shén* carries many inherited abilities and potentials, and the acquired *shén* depends on those attributes. For example, the acquired *shén* carries out postnatal reading and learning activities, but it is the initiating *shén* that gives us the ability to read and learn.

Because the *shén qì* homes to the heart, the governor of acquired *shén* conscious awareness is known as the heart-*shén*. Once the baby is born, the acquired *shén* develops and matures through accumulating and processing its own experiences. As 'sovereign ruler' (君主 *jūn zhǔ*), the heart-*shén* coordinates the five postnatal *shén*. The 'five *shén*' (五神 *wǔ shén*) arise and differentiate from the initiating *shén* and each of them contributes in specific ways to our postnatal activities and abilities. Collectively, these are the acquired *shén*.

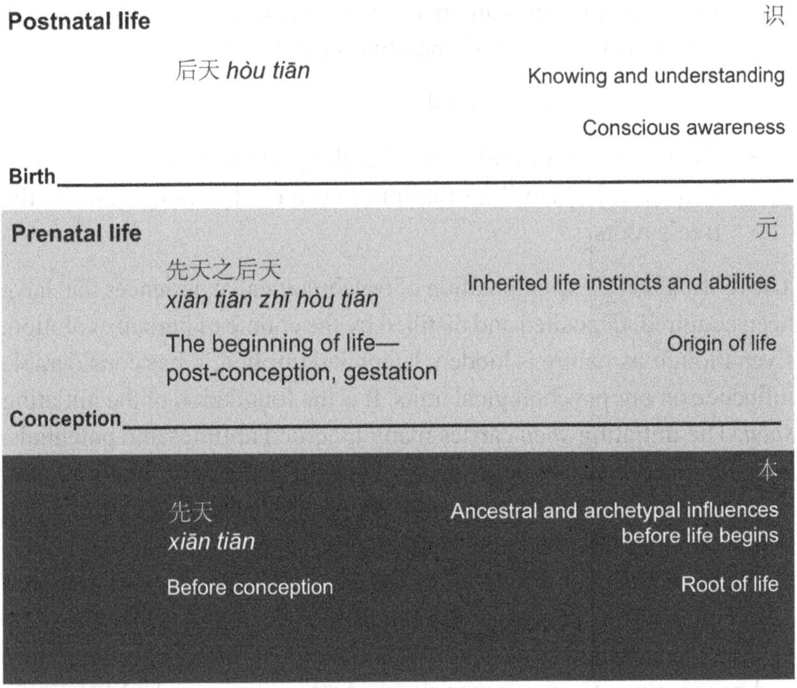

Postnatal life   识

后天 *hòu tiān*   Knowing and understanding

Conscious awareness

Birth_____

Prenatal life   元

先天之后天
xiān tiān zhī hòu tiān   Inherited life instincts and abilities

The beginning of life—   Origin of life
post-conception, gestation

Conception_____

本

先天   Ancestral and archetypal influences
xiān tiān   before life begins

Before conception   Root of life

Figure 3.4: The three aspects of shén—*temporal and formative stages*

Figure 3.4 shows the three aspects of *shén* in terms of their formative stages, and their relationships according to the pre- and postnatal stages of human life. Prenatal life is shown in the lower part of the figure, and postnatal life in the upper part. This representation alludes to the hidden roots of a tree below ground and its visible branches and leaves above ground.

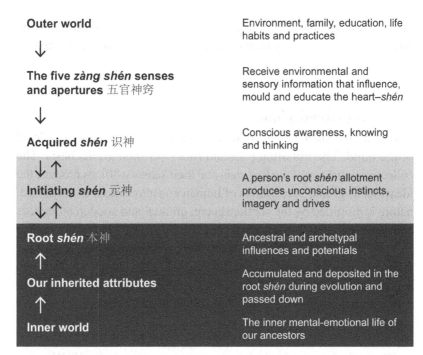

Outer world ↓	Environment, family, education, life habits and practices
The five *zàng shén* senses and apertures 五官神窍 ↓	Receive environmental and sensory information that influence, mould and educate the heart–*shén*
Acquired *shén* 识神	Conscious awareness, knowing and thinking
↓ ↑ **Initiating *shén*** 元神 ↓ ↑	A person's root *shén* allotment produces unconscious instincts, imagery and drives
Root *shén* 本神 ↑	Ancestral and archetypal influences and potentials
Our inherited attributes ↑	Accumulated and deposited in the root *shén* during evolution and passed down
Inner world	The inner mental-emotional life of our ancestors

Figure 3.5: The three aspects of shén—*developmental and interactive relationships*

Figure 3.5 shows the developmental and interactive relationships between the three aspects of *shén*. The postnatal activities of the heart-*shén* are based on the attributes of its prenatal root and origin, and the experiences of our life journey accumulate and shape our disposition and inner life. At the same time, it seems that the root *shén* can be affected by some exceptional postnatal life experiences. When the *Divine Pivot* Treatise 49 says that: '*Shén* accumulates in the heart, it knows the past and the present,'[92] it is indicating that some life experiences are so strong that they can deeply affect the *shén* over time and beyond this life. Some life experiences that make a deep impression on the acquired *shén* may be deposited in the root *shén* and transmitted to the next generation. The Chinese say these kinds of events and influences are 'engraved in the bones and imprinted on the heart.'

The importance of the three aspects and their relationships for clinical practice relates to understanding our patients' conditions and prognosis. TCM sees DNA and chromosomal disorders, for example, as originating at the level of the root and initiating *jīng shén*. Mental and emotional disorders may be due to acquired postnatal conditions

---

92 《灵枢·五色》: 积神于心，以知往今 *Líng shū, Wǔ sè: 'Jī shén yú xīn, yǐ zhī wǎng jīn'*

or traumas, or they may arise due to predisposing constitutional and inherited factors, or they may occur and develop due to a combination of both.

识神 Acquired *shén*

The 'acquired *shén*' (识神 *shí shén*) is the observable, conscious level of the mind. The initiating (元) and root (本) *shén* are its basis. The collective activities of the five *shén* and their sensory offices produce the ideas, feelings and perceptions of human consciousness. Its 'acquired' nature is moulded by the subtle, severe, gradual and sudden influences and experiences of our postnatal life. The *shí shén* (识神) is also called *shén shí* (神识). *Shén shí* is the heart-*shén*'s recognition, understanding and acquisition of knowledge and skills. Although *shén shí* recognition and understanding are performed by the activities of all five *shén* and their associated senses, it is the heart-*shén* that coordinates and manages cognition and conscious awareness. This means that everything we do depends on the heart-*shén* (Qu and Garvey 2006).

Through the acquired *shén* we gain our sense of self. We gain awareness of our inner and outer worlds through its thinking, sensing, knowing and responding. Our sentient mind is able to know and feel our inner world, to perceive and recognize the outer world through the five senses, and to comprehend the connections between our external environment and inner self. The acquired *shén* (识神) receives sensory information from inside and outside the body via our sense organs and body tissues and consists of these sensory perceptions, feelings and thoughts. Postnatal sensory and cognitive activities begin to arise as the physical body is formed: the acquired *shén* is awakened by its reactions to the impressions it receives from the senses. The five *yīn* visceral systems (五藏/五脏 *wǔ zàng*) develop during gestation, forming the heart, liver, lung, spleen and kidney.[93] As they do, the initiating *shén qì* homes to the heart and differentiates into the 'five *shén*' (五神 *wǔ shén*), the *shén*, *hún*, *pò*, *yì* and *zhì*.[94]

As the heart, liver, lungs, spleen and kidneys take form, they are able to lodge each of the five *shén*. This process gradually allows the unborn baby to perceive sensory information through the mother and

---

93 心 *xīn*, 肝 *gān*, 肺 *fèi*, 脾 *pí* and 肾 *shèn*
94 神 *shén*, 魂 *hún*, 魄 *pò*, 意 *yì* and 志 *zhì*

her environment. The developing *zàng* visceral systems and five *shén* allow the unborn baby to gradually absorb some sensory influences and begin to understand the environment around them. This means that both the initiating *shén* and the developing acquired *shén* contribute to our prenatal *shén* during gestation. After birth, the acquired *shén* develops and matures through accumulating and processing its own experiences.

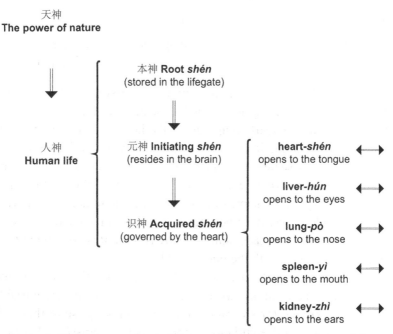

Figure 3.6: The three aspects of shén, *and the five postnatal* zàng shén

[After birth], the [initiating *shén*] dwells between and behind the eyes, and the conscious [*shén*] dwells below in the heart… This heart is dependent on the outside world. If one does not eat for a day even, it feels extremely uncomfortable. If it hears something terrifying it throbs; if it hears something enraging it stops; if it is faced with death it becomes sad; if it sees something beautiful it is dazzled. (Wilhelm 1984, p.25)

In TCM, '神 *shén*' refers to postnatal life and conscious awareness. Postnatal conscious awareness, the acquired *shén*, encompasses the five *shén* that arise from the undifferentiated initiating *shén*. Conscious awareness, knowing and understanding occurs due to the heart-*shén*'s coordination, recognition and analysis of the five *shén* and their sensory perceptions. Therefore, TCM also uses '神 *shén*' more specifically, to refer to the heart-*shén*. The heart-*shén* governs human intelligence. It makes us awake, alert and responsive during the day; at night, it becomes inactive and returns to its lodging in the heart.

心神 *The heart-shén*
The *Divine Pivot* Treatise 54 states that:

> As the five *zàng* develop [in-utero], the *shén qì* settles in the heart, the *hún* and *pò* are formed, and thereupon human life is accomplished.[95]

The '*shén qì*' (神气) in this quotation is at first the initiating *shén*. During gestation, *shén qì* is assigned to the heart-*shén* (心神) as it takes up its place in the heart *zàng*. Part of the heart *shén qì* also takes its place to reside in the liver and lung *zàng* as the *hún* (魂) and *pò* (魄) respectively. These three, the *shén*, *hún* and *pò*, are essential for normal human life. As the *shén qì* differentiates, the developing foetus begins to feel and experience some of its environmental influences. It may be that the *Divine Pivot* does not mention spleen-*yì* (意) and kidney-*zhì* (志) at this stage because, until the baby is born, it is not able to think or connect directly with the outer world.

Even at birth, spleen-*yì* and kidney-*zhì* activities are minimal because the infant's middle *qì* and kidney *qì* are immature and unstable. Babies are known for sleeping rather than thinking, so at this early stage, five-phase differentiation emphasizes the heart-*shén*, liver-*hún* and lung-*pò* activities, which shows how important these resources are for early survival and development. While sensory perceptions and responses arise relatively quickly, the cognitive processes involved in recollection, analysis, judgment and memory (the spleen and kidney/*yì* and *zhì* mental functions) develop more slowly over a number of years.

After birth, the baby begins to experience, recognize and recall by looking, touching, hearing, and so on. At the same time, the five *zàng shén*[96] gradually establish their relationships with the 'five sensory organs and their apertures.'[97] Sense apertures are our windows to

---

95   《灵枢·天年》：五藏已成，神气舍心，魂魄必俱，乃成为人。*Líng shū, Tiān nián: 'Wǔ zàng yǐ chéng, shén qì shě xīn, hún pò bì jù, nǎi chéng wéi rén'*
96   五藏神 *wǔ zàng shén*—the heart-*shén*, liver-*hún*, lung-*pò*, spleen-*yì*, kidney-*zhì*
97   五官神窍 *wǔ guān shén qiào*—the tongue, eyes, nose, mouth and ears

the external world. Through these, the baby's faculties of thinking, feeling and remembering begin gradually to receive and interpret sensory information independently from the mother. The role of the senses, to receive and interpret the external world, is crucial to how we experience life.

The heart-*shén* governs human consciousness, and importantly for TCM practice, its conscious awareness incorporates physical, mental and emotional activities and responses. It is the heart-*shén* that manages our emotions and desires, and experiences love, generosity, happiness, attachment, aversion and hatred. Its function in healthy physiological and mental/emotional activities can be observed in a person's healthy complexion, bright eyes, physical agility and coherent speech.

In Chinese medicine, the heart-*shén* is the sovereign ruler. At night, it settles in the heart, and during the day it makes us awake, alert and responsive. It manages the acquired *shén*'s sensory perceptions and cognitive activities and thereby rules human consciousness and cognition. It receives, coordinates and analyzes sensory information from all five *zàng shén*: the heart-*shén* itself, the liver-*hún*, lung-*pò*, spleen-*yì* and kidney-*zhì*.

* * *

The three aspects of *shén* explain how our inherited *shén* characteristics are not only from our immediate parents but from many, many generations of ancestors. Like a seed or egg, the root *shén* has its own vitality within. It resides in the kidney-lifegate and its evolutionary information enables human survival. The root *shén* constitutes the inherited source of our mental and emotional life, and the source *qì* that arises from the lifegate is its diffuse influence of ancestral, parental and constitutional life information. Postnatal conscious awareness and the activities of knowing and understanding are impossible without the prenatal root, the source and origin of the *shén*'s potentials and abilities.

When a new life arises, this is the initiating *shén*. The initiating *shén* instigates life, and after birth it resides in the brain. It carries evolutionary and basic life abilities (such as breathing and heartbeat), instinctual and survival abilities and drives (such as eating and sex), and our sensory, survival and language abilities. Together, the root and initiating *shén* are the prenatal aspects of *shén* that guide our postnatal human life, its development and direction.

The abilities and potentials of the acquired *shén* are based on the initiating and root *shén*. After birth, these inner inherited resources are developed, moulded and extended by our environment, family, education and opportunities. The acquired *shén* is a complex of the influences and experiences of postnatal sensory awareness and perceptions, and the heart-*shén*'s analysis and coordination of the sensory information received by the five *zàng shén*. Education, self-cultivation and other acquired *shén* activities allow us to develop and extend the attributes we have inherited from many generations and, indeed, from all our biological ancestors.

When we consider the influence of the root of the *shén*, it is impossible to imagine the complexity of each person's psychological characteristics, or the countless variety of formative events and memories. If it were possible to know the many millions of significant, 'carved in the bone' life experiences that our ancestors endured, we could begin to develop a more longitudinal and integrated study of the formation, feedback, response and development of the human psyche.

Chapter 4

Mind and Emotions

Chinese medicine's theories of the mind (神志 *shén zhì*) and emotions (情志 *qíng zhì*) are the basis of TCM psychology today. *Shén zhì* theory is drawn largely from the *Divine Pivot* Treatise 8 and from other sections of the *Inner Canon*. These clearly record the *shén* resources and relationships that contribute to sensory perception, analysis, consciousness and cognition. During gestation, the *shén qì* homes to the heart from where it coordinates the five *shén*: *shén, hún, pò, yì* and *zhì*. As the foetus develops, the five *shén* begin to contribute in specific ways to sentient life. Together, their collective activities are the acquired *shén* with the heart as eminent ruler. *Shén zhì* theory explains the nature of the five *shén* and their governance of and relationships with our sensory faculties, body structures, *qì* substances and emotional life. The orderly activities of the five *shén* produce the knowing and understanding of our conscious awareness, the acquired *shén*.

The *Divine Pivot* Treatise 8 sets out the activities of the five *shén*, their reception and analysis of sensory information, and their interdependent functions creating human consciousness, intelligence and cognitive ability. The number five signals that five-phase correspondences supply the theoretical underpinning and that all its relational qualities apply. The middle section of the *Divine Pivot* Treatise 8, and elsewhere in the *Inner Canon*, explains the relationships between the *zàng*, their *shén*, cognitive activities and emotional responses. The latter part of Treatise 8 establishes the relationship between the *zàng shén* and their *qì* substances. In Line 100, for instance:

The liver stores blood, and the blood holds the *hún*.[98]

---

98 《灵枢·本神》：肝藏血，血舍魂。*Líng shū, Běn shén: 'Gān cáng xuè, xuè shè hún'*

Normal *shén zhì* activities and *qíng zhì* responses therefore depend on harmonious relationships between the five *shén* (五神 *wǔ shén*) and with their respective *yīn* visceral systems (五藏 *wǔ zàng*), sense organs (五官 *wǔ guān*) and body tissues (五体 *wǔ tǐ*). All five body/ mind systems provide specific kinds of sensory data and the heart-*shén* receives, coordinates and analyzes this complex stream of information. Sensory perceptions begin with the clarity of the information we receive through the sensory offices, and the reliability of our perceptions then depends on correct recognition, analysis and interpretation of that information.

These relationships are essential for understanding the patho-mechanisms producing the signs and symptoms of mental and emotional illness. For example, the heart-*shén* governs the tongue, speech and communication, and happiness is the emotion associated with the heart. This is why speaking can relieve pressure on the heart and talking with friends can be recommended therapeutically. The spleen-*yì* receives and differentiates the five tastes, the kidney-*zhì* receives aural information, and the lung-*pò*, tactile and olfactory information. The liver opens to the eyes so the *hún* participates in the reception and transmission of visual information. Because it governs the sinews and the movement of joints, the liver-*hún* also transmits sensory information regarding movement, balance and proprioception. Because anger is associated with the liver, excessive or prolonged angry responses harm the liver-*hún*, its corresponding sensory functions and body tissues.

神志学说 *Shén zhì* theory

'*Shén zhì* theory'[99] explains the principles behind Chinese medicine psychology and its view of human conscious awareness. *Shén zhì* (神志) is an abbreviation for the *shén, hún, pò, yì* and *zhì*, and is another name for the 'mind.' *Shén zhì* theory is based on the five *zàng shén*. Their governance of certain aspects of our mental and emotional life, sensory faculties, body tissues, visceral systems and physiological activities, follows the five-phase (五行 *wǔ xíng*) framework of correspondence and relationship.

Table 4.1 shows the immediate areas of influence and responsibility for the five *zàng*. The lung, for instance, lodges the *pò* and opens to the

---

99 神志学说 *shén zhì xué shuō*

nose to receive olfactory information. The body tissues governed by the lung are the skin and soft body hair. Because these are important sensory structures sensitive to the external environment, we include tactile perceptions in the lung column. The heart *zàng* lodges the *shén* and opens to the tongue. In this case, the function of the tongue is that of the moving part of the voice, so when the heart-*shén* is healthy, speech is fluent and communication is appropriate. In the *Elementary Questions* Treatise 8, the heart-*shén*'s role is that of the head of state. In the *Divine Pivot* Treatise 8, the heart-*shén* coordinates sensory information to analyze and manage all external and internal matters. It is the nature of the *shén zhì* that these processes are accomplished instantly.

Table 4.1: *Shén zhì* **comprises the five**
zàng shén, **their senses and body tissues**

神志 *shén zhì*					
五藏 *wǔ zàng*	心 heart	肝 liver	肺 lung	脾 spleen	肾 kidney
五神 *wǔ shén*	神 *shén*	魂 *hún*	魄 *pò*	意 *yì*	志 *zhì*
五官 *wǔ guān*	舌 *shé* tongue	目 *mù* eyes	鼻 *bí* nose	口 *kǒu* mouth	耳 *ěr* ears
receives sensory information	speaking, receives and manages all sensory information	眼识 *yǎn* *shí* vision	鼻识 *bí* *shí* smell, 身识 *shēn shí* touch	舌识 *shé* *shí* taste	耳识 *ěr* *shí* hearing
五体 *wǔ tǐ*	脉 *mài* vessels	筋 *jīn* sinews	皮 *pí* skin	肉 *ròu* flesh	骨 *gǔ* bones

The associations shown in Table 4.1 inform Chinese diagnostic observation and reasoning, and there are many more. For instance, the heart governs the blood and the vessels, and the heart blood holds the *shén*. Therefore, the orderly or disorderly state of the heart-*shén* is observable in the complexion. In addition, the heart manifests in the eyes, opens to the tongue and governs the act of speaking, and laughing is a heart sound. Therefore social, behavioral and communication skills provide a clear indication of the condition of the heart-*shén* and its management of mental and emotional perceptions and responses.

When spoken and emotional communication are lucid and appropriate, we know how best to manage and respond to stimulus, events and circumstances; we know what we should or should not do or say, when to laugh and when not to. The patient with heart-*shén* illness patterns may experience disturbances involving speech, consciousness, inappropriate moods and laughter. Disorders can include disorganized or incoherent speech, dyslogia, aphasia, delirium, psychosis, mania or coma. Detailed understanding of these relationships allows us to apply *shén zhì* theory to the illness manifestations recorded in the Chinese medicine classics. *Shén zhì* theory applies equally well to the analysis and interpretation of the signs and symptoms of mental disorder as they present in our clinics today.

To produce human consciousness, the harmonious interactions of all five *shén*, their associated viscera, sense organs and body tissues process visual, olfactory, taste, tactile, auditory and other perceived information. The smooth analysis and synthesis of information, the ability to respond, recall and communicate, the accomplished elegance of human consciousness, indicate orderly *shén zhì* activities.

五神学说 Five shén theory

In Chinese medicine, *shén zhì* comprises the *shén*, *hún*, *pò*, *yì*, *zhì* and their distinctive array of mental and sensory abilities, the intelligence, insight, focused attention and memory that are characteristic of human life (人神). During gestation, the foetus's life resources develop and the body form takes shape. From the inherited *jīng shén* resources, the *zàng* and *shén* differentiate and develop. According to early Chinese thinking, these processes follow *yīn/yáng* (阴阳) and five-phase (五行) correspondences. The differentiation of the five postnatal *shén* mirrors the generation of the five *zàng*, and the *Inner Canon* describes how the *yīn* visceral systems nourish and protect the most *yáng* and ethereal aspects of human life, the five *shén*.

In the *Elementary Questions* Treatise 4, Qí Bó explains that each of the *zàng* can receive and collect sensory information because they hold the *jīng*-essence. Treatise 4 goes on to say that, 'The South, red colour; enters and communicates with the heart; [the heart] opens to the ears, and stores essence.'[100] Whereas, Treatise 5 states that the kidney *zàng* opens to the ears. *Shén zhì* theory explains that we need both the kidney's *jīng*-essence and the heart-*shén*'s analysis to receive and understand auditory information.

- **The 神 *shén* resides in the heart.** We perceive and respond to the external world every waking moment via a steady stream of sensory information. Normal heart-*shén* activities ensure that our conscious awareness, cognitive functions, communication and emotional responses are orderly and clear. When they are, the five *shén*, their *zàng* viscera, body tissues and senses function harmoniously, and our body–mind activities are responsive and appropriate.

- **The 魂 *hún* resides in the liver.** The liver governs the sinews, opens to the eyes, stores the blood, and liver blood holds the *hún*. Therefore, the liver-*hún* participates in the perception of visual information and in the movement and balance of the body, its flexibility, strength and agility.

- **The 魄 *pò* resides in the lung.** The lung holds the *pò*, opens to the nose and corresponds to the skin and body hair. The lung-*pò* therefore participates in perceiving sensory information via the nose and skin; it is sensitive to the environment around the body, registering cold and heat and helping us to avoid danger. According to Zhāng Jièbīn's *Classified Canon*,[101] 'The function of the *pò* is to enable the body to move and perform its function; pain and itching are felt by it.'

- **The 意 *yì* resides in the spleen.** The spleen-*yì* forms ideas, focuses thinking and carries out the initial processing of sensations and perceptions. Its recalled experience and knowledge are essential to the heart-*shén*'s processing of sensory information. Together, they accomplish first-stage information processing and understanding.

---

100 《素问·金匮真言论篇》：南方赤色，入通于心，开窍于耳，藏精于心。
   Sù wèn, Jīn guì zhēn yán lùn piān: 'Nán fāng chì sè, rù tōng yú xīn, kāi qiào yú ěr, cáng jīng yú xīn'
101 《类经》 *Lèi jīng*, 1624

- **The 志 *zhì* resides in the kidney.** The kidney governs 'seal and store' (封藏 *fēng cáng*). The kidney opens to the ear so the kidney-*zhì* participates in the reception of auditory information. The kidney stores *jīng*-essence and in the same way the kidney-*zhì* completes the storage of information. The kidney-*zhì*'s memory, skill and determination provide a breadth and depth of understanding that allow us the possibilities of 'ideals and ambition' (志向 *zhì xiàng*), and the potential to attain wisdom and intelligence. All these features rely on the kidney's storage of *jīng*-essence.

情志学说 *Qíng zhì* theory

Chinese medicine's theory of the emotions is very straightforward. Emotional responses are observable manifestations that come from the functional (*qì*) aspects of the five *zàng shén*. In the *Elementary Questions* Treatise 5[102] says:

> The five *zàng* transform the five *qì*, which manifests the five kinds of emotions, joy, anger, sadness, pensiveness and fear.

In this life, our character and disposition are reflected in our heart-*shén*'s governance of emotions. When the *shén* is happy and optimistic, the emotions are relaxed and positive. The *Divine Pivot* Treatise 8 sets out the relationships between the *zàng*, their *qì* influences and substances, and it describes how excessive emotions disrupt them. For example, unresolved worry and too much thinking binds and weakens the middle *qì* and harms the spleen-*yì*.

情志 *Qíng zhì* means 'emotions,' 'memory' and 'dispositions,' and '*qíng zhì* theory'[103] is an important part of *shén zhì* theory. In 1602, Wáng Kěntáng introduced the term '*shén zhì* disease'[104] as an illness category where mental symptoms are the significant features. Similarly, emotion-related disorders[105] only became a distinct illness category from the late Ming dynasty when Zhāng Jièbīn (1562–1639) introduced their grouping into what we now call the *qíng zhì* disorders.

---

102 《素问·阴阳应象大论》 *Sù wèn, Yīn yáng yīng xiàng dà lùn* 人有五藏化五气，以生喜怒悲忧恐 *rén yǒu wǔ zàng huà wǔ qì, yǐ shēng xǐ nù bēi yōu kǒng*
103 情志学说 *qíng zhì xué shuō*
104 神志病 *shén zhì bìng*
105 情志病 *qíng zhì bìng*

Many of the illnesses Zhāng assigned to this category can be found in the classic literature, such as the plum stone throat syndrome, and we discuss some of them in Part 2.

Strictly speaking, emotion-related illnesses are not psychiatric, mood or mental disorders; they are illnesses that originate from 'internal injury due to excessive emotions'[106] (Zhang 2007). 'Internal injury' simply means that emotion-related disorders are closely related to the internal viscera and their *qì* activities. Because the emotions affect internal *qì* activities, excessive emotional responses disrupt orderly movements and transformations and cause illness.

Chinese medicine's five emotions (五志 *wǔ zhì*) are: joy, anger, sadness, pensiveness and fear. The seven emotions (七情 *qī qíng*) add worry and fright. By combining worry with pensiveness, and fear with fright, we can align the seven emotions with the five minds (五 志 *wǔ zhì*). 情 *Qíng* and 志 *zhì* are frequently used together, as they are for Chinese medicine's emotions theory (情志学说). While *qíng* are observable emotional responses, *zhì* are more latent, underlying states, our temperament and emotional memory. The emotions have both normal and pathological effects on the *qì* depending on their appropriateness, intensity and duration, and our ability to move freely into and out of our emotional states.

Not only are emotional responses observable manifestations of *qì*, we can actually feel their immediate impact in terms of *qì* movement. According to the *Inner Canon*:

- Happiness and joy relax the *qì*.

- Anger causes the *qì* to rise.

- Sadness and grief weaken and deplete the *qì*.

- Pensiveness and excess thinking cause the *qì* to knot and congeal.

- Worry and obsession slow the *qì*.

- Fear causes the *qì* to descend.

- Fright causes the *qì* to become chaotic.

The *Inner Canon* sets out the relationships between the *zàng shén* and the emotions. Not all the *Inner Canon* texts agree exactly on this;

---

106 情志内伤 *qíng zhì nèi shāng*

for example, some associate worry rather than sadness with the lung. We tabulate the *Inner Canon*'s emotion and *zàng shén* associations alongside their known effects on *qì* movement in Table 4.2.

Table 4.2: The emotions, their associated *zàng shén* and effects on the *qì*

Emotion	The disposition of the...	Its effect on *qì* movement
喜 *xǐ* **joy**	heart-*shén*	relaxes the *qì* (excess causes the *qì* to become sluggish and damages the heart)
怒 *nù* **anger**	liver-*hún*	ascends the *qì* (excess causes ascending *yáng* and damages the liver)
忧 *yōu* **worry**	affects all the *zàng*, especially the lung-*pò* and spleen-*yì*	slows the *qì* (excess slows and depletes the *qì*)
思 *sī* **pensiveness, thinking**	spleen-*yì*	slows the *qì* (excess binds and knots the *qì* and weakens the spleen)
悲 *bēi* **grief, sadness**	lung-*pò*	weakens the *qì* (excess depletes the *qì* and damages the lung)
恐 *kǒng* **fear**	kidney-*zhì*	descends the *qì* (excess causes the *qì* to sink and damages the kidney)
惊 *jīng* **fright**	affects all the *zàng*, especially the heart-*shén*, liver-*hún* and kidney-*zhì*	the *qì* becomes disordered and chaotic

The *zàng*-emotion associations mean that emotional changes influence the body interior in predictable ways. For example, anger especially affects the liver; and when angry responses are excessive and prolonged, there is an interior climate of, and tendency towards, *qì* rising. This disrupts the *qì* mechanism. The liver loses its ability to spread the *qì* and maintain free, unobstructed movement; excess *qì* rising disrupts the orderly exchange of ascending and descending; and because the liver is a *yáng* viscera, the unsmooth and rising *qì* tends to transform into pathogenic heat. Over time, prolonged anger or an angry temperament changes the liver *zàng*, and then the disordered liver easily produces more anger and resentment, rising heat, *qì* constraint and internal disorder.

Inter-relationships

The complexity and finesse of the acquired *shén*'s conscious awareness is the result of the harmonious activities of the five *zàng shén*, their senses and body tissues, and the movement and transformation of the essence, *qì*, blood and fluids. Each of the *zàng shén*, their *qì* substances, influences and emotions, their *yīn* and *yáng* and five-phase qualities must cooperate harmoniously. Their integrated activities and interactions accomplish human life and enable us to act in the world. To effectively treat mental and emotional disorders, Chinese medicine practitioners must develop a detailed understanding of their individual characteristics and physiological relationships.

The *Divine Pivot* Treatise 8 describes many of the relationships that contribute to feelings and sensation, analysis, cognition and consciousness. To convey states of mental disruption and cognitive disintegration, Treatise 8 names disorders in terms of these relationships, such as when the '*hún* and *pò* are scattered' or they 'fly upwards,' or the '*jīng, shén, hún* and *pò* are scattered,' or the '*zhì* and *yì* are confused and disordered.' Part 2's discussion of disorders and treatment strategies begins with some of these early disruptions.

Line 103 of Treatise 8 says: 'The spleen stores the *yíng* and *yíng* lodges the *yì*.'[107] **Heart-*shén* and spleen-*yì*** reflection and analysis depend on the spleen's formation and storage of 'nutrient' (營 *yíng*) *qì*. When we are tired and hungry, *yíng qì* is depleted and this causes our thinking to become muddled and slow. Similarly, the reason that someone with heart blood and spleen *qì* vacuity complains of slow thinking and poor memory is that their '**nutrient and blood**' (營血 *yíng–xuè*) is depleted. In cases of sudden and severe blood loss, the spleen can no longer lodge the *yì* and the patient goes into shock. In serious cases, the *shén* also flees and they lose consciousness. The unconscious patient is not capable of sensing, processing or responding.

Together, the spleen-*yì* and heart-*shén* accomplish first-stage perception and analysis of ideas. The kidney-*zhì* and heart-*shén* relationship enables more sophisticated processing and depth of understanding. According to Line 27 in Treatise 8 (given above in Chapter 1), when spleen-*yì* activities are retained as part of the mind's stored experience, the kidney-*zhì*'s 'seal and store' (封藏 *fēng cáng*)

---

107 《灵枢·本神》: 脾藏营，营舍意。 *Líng shū, Běn shén: 'Pí cāng yíng, yíng shě yì'*

function performs this. Physiologically, the kidney preserves the pre- and postnatal *jīng*-essence, and psychologically it preserves our memories, including our emotional memories. The *jīng*-essence provides the material basis for kidney activities, so when the essence is abundant, the kidney's seal and store functions, including its memory function, are strong.

The kidney's seal and store functions distil and preserve the results of **heart-*shén* and kidney-*zhì*** activities, and depleted **kidney *jīng*** disrupts their relationship. When the *shén–zhì* relationship is disordered, the patient is likely to have memory problems. They may have hearing problems, because the kidney opens to the ears. So, for example, it is common for the elderly to experience some degree of memory impairment and/or auditory deficit corresponding to the decline of *jīng*-essence that normally occurs with age. Similarly, *shén–zhì* disorder is typical in dementia patients with failing memory and multiple cognitive deficits. In severe cases of heart-*shén* and kidney-*zhì* disorder there may be amnesia or auditory hallucinations. The combined functions of the **heart-*shén*, spleen-*yì* and kidney-*zhì*** contribute to awareness and **memory**—the *shén* for reception and analysis, the *yì* to assist processing, and the *zhì* for storage. The creation and storage of memories are cared for by the three *zàng* most closely associated with the three treasures (精气神 *jīng qì shén*) and our ancestral resources.

The *Divine Pivot* Treatise 8 establishes the importance of the **shén–hún** relationship in Line 23: 'That which faithfully comes and goes following the *shén*, is the *hún*.'[108] The *shén–hún* 'coming and going' (往来 *wǎng lái*) facilitates the communication between internal (body and mind) and external (environmental) conditions. This is an area of subtle exchange that depends on the *shén–hún*'s ability to move freely between the two. Visual perception exemplifies their relationship: when the *shén* wants to look at something, the *hún* follows and focuses immediately on the object of attention. The heart-*shén* receives visual information via the liver-*hún*-eyes, engages recall and ascertains meaning.

When the *shén–hún* are orderly and harmonious, their coming and going is swift and light, barely registering in our conscious mind.

---

108 《灵枢 · 本神》：随神往来者謂之魂。 *Líng shū, Běn shén: 'Suí shén wǎng lái zhě wèi zhī hún'*

Their connectedness allows us to realize the more subtle qualities of knowing and understanding. The *Zhuāng Zǐ* Chapter 2 calls it the 'capacity for unknowing,' a kind of 'spirit brightness' (*shén míng*) or intelligence, and says that the *hún* often makes these connections and relationships during sleep.[109]

If the *hún* fails to follow the *shén*, the body form and *shén* are no longer unified. The person's eyes are blank because the liver-*hún* cannot correctly transmit what it is seeing to the heart-*shén*, and the heart-*shén* cannot assess the matters being perceived by the liver-*hún*. This is why in Chinese medicine we say that the liver stores blood, liver blood nourishes the eyes and holds the *hún*, heart blood houses the *shén*, the *shén* and *hún* always follow each other when we are awake, and the eyes are the window of the soul.

Shén zhì activities depend on the harmonious relationships between the five *shén* and their respective viscera, *qì* substances, tissues and senses. For instance, the liver stores blood, the liver blood holds the *hún* and the liver opens to the eyes. So, the liver-*hún*'s ability to receive visual information relies on the liver blood nourishing its sensory structures and apertures. Moreover, the liver blood nourishes the sinews, so the liver-*hún* senses and enables bodily movement, flexibility and awareness.

The heart and liver's physiological responsibilities for governing and storing the blood support their *shén qì* functions. The *shén–hún* relationship, their orderly going and coming, is nourished by the **liver and heart blood**, and supported by a peaceful mind. The coming and going of the *shén* and *hún* therefore is both a physiological and psychological state. Their relationship is disturbed by agitation, pathogenic heat, emotional upset and depleted blood, and when the *hún* fails to follow the *shén*, this leads to mental disorder.

The balance between the ***hún* and *pò*** relies on their complementary relationships with **blood and *qì***, and with the ***shén* and *jīng*-essence**, respectively. Line 24 of the *Divine Pivot* Treatise 8 describes the *pò*

---

109 《莊子，齊物論》：其寐也魂交，其覺也形開，與接為構，日以心鬭。*Zhuāng Zi, Qi wù lùn: 'Qí mèi yě hún jiāo, qí jué yě xíng kāi, yǔ jiē wèi gòu, rì yǐ xīn dòu.'* (Chapter 2) 'The Adjustment of Controversies': 'When we sleep, the *shén–hún* communicates with [what is external and internal to us]; when we awake, the body is set free and intelligence becomes active'

and *jīng*-essence connection: 'That which enters and leaves together with the essence, is the *pò*.'[110]

With the first breath, the lung-*pò* becomes active. The ***jīng-pò*** 'entering and exiting' (出入 *chū rù*) relationship refers to breathing, absorption and excretion, birth and death. From birth and until the end of our physical existence, the *jīng-pò* sees to the day-to-day direction and maintenance of life—the breath entering and exiting, assimilation and elimination. The lung opens to the nose, corresponds to the skin and body hair, and is sensitive to the environment around the body, registering cold and heat.

Depleted **lung *qì*** or ***jīng*-essence** compromise *jīng-pò* entering and exiting and lung-*pò* activities, and are likely to disrupt ***shén-pò*** cognitive, sensory activities and emotional responses. Signs and symptoms of *shén-pò* disharmony include disordered or abnormal sensations, for example olfactory or tactile hypersensitivity, dysesthesia, paresthesia, anosmia and olfactory hallucinations. Depleted *jīng* also affects the *pò*'s role in physical movement, and falls are common in the elderly as they lose their strength and dexterity.

Diabetic neuropathy is another illustration of these physiological relationships. The term 'consumption thirst' (消渴 *xiāo kě*) was first mentioned in the *Inner Canon* (*c.* 100 BCE), and then in the *Essential Prescriptions of the Golden Cabinet* (*c.* 220 CE) in Line 13.4. Nowadays, it is often suggested as an equivalent TCM disease name for diabetes. In Chinese medicine, the *xiāo kě* patient experiences a loss of *jīng*-essence because of (diabetic) polyuria, which in turn is due to the kidney *qì* 'failing to hold.' Polyuria worsens the loss of *qì* and *jīng*-essence, and the disruption to the *jīng-pò* relationship leads to sensation disorders such as numbness and peripheral neuritis. While dispersion thirst, depleted essence, diabetes, polyuria and peripheral neuritis are not symptoms of mental illness, the Chinese medicine view emphasizes the functional links between the *zàng fǔ* and their associated *qì* substances, body tissues, sense organs and *shén*. Disordered sensations such as diabetic neuropathy are an example of *shén-pò* (mental-sensory) disharmony, and demonstrate the *jīng-pò* physiological relationship.

In the *Elementary Questions* Treatise 8, the heart is the supreme commander and the heart-*shén* plays the leading role in the correct

---

110 《灵枢 · 本神》： 並精而出入者謂之魄。 *Líng shū, Běn shén: 'Bìng jīng ér chū rù zhě wèi zhī pò'*

functioning of our conscious awareness. Disruption with any aspect or at any stage of the five *shén* activities (including their visceral–sensory–body tissue functions, emotional activities and interactions) can impair the heart-*shén* and its brightness (神明 *shén míng*). Conversely, normal heart-*shén* activities ensure consciousness and cognition are clear and rational. When the five *shén*, viscera, senses and body tissues function harmoniously with *shén míng* brightness and clarity, body and mind activities are responsive and appropriate.

Constitution and personality

TCM basic theory explains the permutations of *qì* and the union of physiology and psychology. According to the *Inner Canon*, the law of *yīn* and *yáng* controls the creation of life, and thereafter it shapes our physical and psychological characteristics. For instance, the *Elementary Questions* Treatise 5 says: '*Yīn* and *Yáng*, the law of heaven and earth, of the universe and all things, the parents of change and transformation, the basis and beginning of life and death, the palace of *shén míng*.'

Chinese medicine's early discussions of human life include ideas about constitutional, personality and body form types and their features. The *Divine Pivot* describes a total of 30 *yīn* and *yáng* and five-phase body and character types; for example, in Treatises 64 and 72.[111] Treatise 72 has a detailed description of five *yīn* and *yáng* types, namely, the major and minor *yīn* (*tàiyīn* and *shǎoyīn*), and the major and minor *yáng* (*tàiyáng* and *shǎoyáng*) types, and those with more even and balanced *yīn–yáng* qualities. Here are some of their character and personality traits:

1. *tàiyīn types:* adhere strongly to the *yīn* and tend to have negative character features. *Yīn* qualities include introverted and passive traits, a quiet disposition and low sex drive. The *Divine Pivot* says they are, 'greedy, opportunistic and lack social competence,' their 'heart is gentle but not open,' and they quietly harbour negative thoughts.

2. *shǎoyīn people:* also adhere to the *yīn* but less so than the *tàiyīn* type. In the *Divine Pivot*, 'Shaoyin people are a little greedy and

---

111 《灵枢 · 阴阳二十五人》 *Líng shū, Yīn yáng èr shí wǔ rén* ('Yīn Yáng and the Twenty-five Human Types'), and 《灵枢 · 通天》 *Líng shū, Tōng tiān* ('Penetrating Heaven')

have the heart of a thief; when others have lost something, they feel that they have gained something; they are envious and lack compassion.'

3. *tàiyáng types:* adhere strongly to the *yáng* and tend to have more positive features. They are inclined to be frugal and contented, and have a strong sexual drive. They are talkative but this is mainly empty talk; they devise grand plans, care little about right and wrong, and in failure they never feel remorse. The *Divine Pivot* describes this character type as, 'making extravagant claims, but lacking the required competence; they act randomly and only in their self-interest.'

4. *shǎoyáng people:* also adhere to the *yáng* but less strongly than *tàiyáng* types. They enjoy social exchanges, are diligent and have a strong sense of self-respect. The *Divine Pivot* says, 'even if they are only minor officials, they still consider themselves something special.'

5. *People whose* yīn *and* yáng *are evenly balanced:* this is the ideal personality type. Their *yīn* and *yáng qì* are relatively harmonious, their words and deeds are appropriate and respectful, and they discuss matters without pressure or force. The *Divine Pivot* says they, 'live in a peaceful, calm environment, with nothing to fear, and nothing to cause enjoyment; they are friendly and fulfil their duties; they never enter into conflict, and wait for changes to occur with time; they accept praise with humility.'

In the *Divine Pivot* Treatise 64, when Huáng Dì asks about the 25 different types of people, Qí Bó uses the five-phase framework to answer. Each phase has a typical constitution and personality type, and is accompanied by four subtypes. First, he distinguishes the five colors of the complexion and their body types. From there he describes their main physical, mental and emotional features and traits. He goes on to discuss the 25 transformations according to the blood and *qì* in the channels and the *yīn* and *yáng* of the outer manifestations. Table 4.3 summarizes the main features of the five primary types.

Table 4.3: The *Inner Canon*'s five-phase personality and body types

Phase and complexion	Physical features and personality traits		
WOOD: green complexion	Small head, long face, broad shoulders and back, straight body, small hands and feet	Intelligent, adept and scheming, anxious, drawn to wise people, easy and amiable	Their abilities are in spring and summer, cannot tolerate autumn and winter, when they tend to fall ill
FIRE: red complexion	Broad teeth, narrow forehead and small head, muscular shoulders and back, well-developed thighs and abdomen, small hands and feet, swing their shoulders and steady steps when walking	Generous with the needy, bold vision, quick mind, modest, sincere, not gullible or naive, but suspicious, hasty, short tempered	Short lifespan and susceptible to sudden death, can tolerate spring and summer but tend to become ill in autumn and winter
EARTH: yellow complexion	Round face, large head, large abdomen, well-developed shoulders and back, beautiful thighs and legs, small hands and feet, fleshy, upper and lower symmetry, steady brisk walking pace	Tranquil and calm, virtuous, generous, honest, sincere, sociable, like helping others, dislike dealing with authority	Able to counter disease in autumn and winter but subject to the beginning of disease in spring and summer
METAL: white complexion	Square face, small head, shoulders, back and abdomen, small hands and feet, skeleton is light, external ankle/heel is prominent, body is nimble and lean	Irascible, anxious, quiet, resolute, they make good officials, honest and steadfast	Can counter disease in autumn and winter but not in spring and summer
WATER: black complexion	Uneven face, large head, angular chin and jaw, small shoulders, large abdomen, active hands and feet, the body sways as they begin walking, long back, long between the waist and coccyx	Unafraid, do not respect others, bullying, base, good swindlers	Death may come from war or in disgrace, able to counter disease in autumn and winter but not in spring or summer

Each of us has different *yīn* and *yáng* qualities and our personality traits reflect these differences. According to TCM psychology, we can all intentionally cultivate our personality and character to correct and balance our *yīn* and *yáng* tendencies. The *Divine Pivot* also points out that practitioners must complement their acupuncture moxibustion treatments with their knowledge of these *yīn* and *yáng* and five-phase states: 'Those in antiquity who knew well how to use needles and moxa, considered the five states,' in order to perfect their treatment methods.

✳ ✳ ✳

Chinese medicine's *shén zhì* theory includes its *qíng zhì* theory and refers to the mental and emotional *qì* activities and relationships of the five *zàng shén*. Together, *shén zhì* and *qíng zhì* theories clarify important distinctions, relationships and characteristics of body/mind physiology and disorder. The main features of TCM's mind and emotions theory, its *zàng shén*, their functions and relationships, are first described in the *Inner Canon*. In the *Inner Canon*, life emerges through the interaction of heaven and earth and microcosmically, at conception, this is the original *yáng* and *yīn* of the parental *jīng*-essences. The original *yīn* and *yáng* transform into the new individual's prenatal *jīng shén*, and are embodied by the three treasures (*jīng qì shén*). These form the basis of postnatal life activities. They produce the body form and the *zàng shén*, and the complex configurations of human life manifest according to five-phase associations.

The body houses the *shén* and the *shén* governs the body form, and *shén zhì* theory explains the relationships and features of body–mind physiology. It describes how each of the five *zàng shén* participate in the experience and analysis of sensory information and the processes of human conscious awareness. When the body and mind are unified, their orderly activities may be observed through the associated emotional responses, sensory perceptions and apertures, bodily structures, appearance and movements of the *zàng shén*. Disintegration occurring in any of their relationships disrupts human life and consciousness.

Healthy *shén zhì* activities can be disturbed by factors from within or outside the body. When *shén zhì* activities are disordered, the body–mind relationships disintegrate and separate, leading to a variety of common and more serious disorders. Chinese medicine analysis identifies the resulting illness categories in terms of *qì* or blood vacuity, *yīn–yáng* imbalance, emotional factors and pathogenic factors such as phlegm, blood stasis, heat, fire and toxins. Disorderly relationships and functions cause body–mind (somato-psychic) disorders, and the signs and symptoms of psychological diseases.

While contemporary psychiatry has investigated and categorized mental disease in great detail, Chinese medicine's pattern and illness identification methods tend to favor broader categories. Therefore, in its narrow sense, *shén zhì* disease[112] refers to serious mental and neurological disease categories such as schizophrenia and epilepsy. More broadly, it refers to the *shén zhì* model, which includes functional and physiological disturbances causing mental and emotional, body and mind, and cognitive and sensory disorders.

Based on early Chinese psychological thought, the *shén zhì* and *qíng zhì* theories provide a reliable framework to examine Chinese medicine's perspective on the 'mind,' and a clear guide for the clinical analysis and management of psychological illnesses today. With careful clinical observation and correct understanding of signs and symptoms, we can clearly recognize the patho-mechanisms of disharmony and accurately identify diagnostic illness patterns. The accurate differentiation of *shén zhì* disorders guides our selection of effective treatment strategies and prescriptions.

---

112 神志病 *shén zhì bìng*

Chapter 5

神明 *Shén Míng*

The cultivation of '*shén* brightness' (神明 *shén míng*) was thought to enhance a person's physical health and longevity, and someone with *shén míng* was said to radiate virtue, clarity and intelligence. At birth, the acquired *shén* is in an uncultured, unenlightened state. A Chinese expression for this state is 'veiled and dark.'[113] As the infant develops and matures, their *shén* gradually evolves towards a state of 'clarity.'[114] The psychological processes involved are lengthy and complex, and in Chinese medicine they are regarded as the development of the acquired *shén* from ignorant and dark to bright and clear. After birth, our progress towards 明 *míng* brightness is the gradual development of analysis, discernment, judgment, rationality[115] and mental–emotional intelligence.

In this chapter, we explore the meaning and contribution of the heart with *shén* brightness for TCM psychology. Early Chinese psychological thinking attributes healthy psychology and personality to the heart as host and ruler of *shén míng*, and many inherited and lifetime factors are thought to contribute to this state. We examine the conditions that influence the brightness and clarity of our heart-*shén* and mental–emotional intelligence. The topic comes from the *Elementary Questions* Treatise 8:

> The heart is the official functioning as ruler. The *shén* [is enlightened towards] brightness (神明) from there. …if the ruler is enlightened, his

---

113 蒙昧 *méng mèi* (obscured and irrational)
114 明晰 *míng xī* (clear and rational)
115 理性 *lǐ xìng* (rationality, reason), an important concept in the Song and Ming dynasties thanks to the work of Zhū Xī (朱熹 1130–1200), Confucian scholar, philosopher and advocate for 格物致知 *gé wù zhì zhī* (the investigation of things)

subjects are safe and peaceful… If the ruler is not enlightened, then the twelve [*zàng fǔ*] officials are in danger.[116]

Treatise 8's analogy of political governance draws attention to the correct fulfilment of the heart's role and its similarities to the role of a nation's head of state. As ruler, the heart governs and coordinates its administration and officials, the *zàng fǔ* visceral systems; and as the host of *míng* brightness, it cultivates illumination, reason and clarity for the nation and its people. In pre-modern China, Daoism, Confucianism and Buddhism identified the influences affecting *shén* brightness and explained the connections between ethical conduct, orderly *qì* movements and transformations, and mind–body health. Orderly, clear and bright heart-*shén* functions have positive ramifications for our person, our *qì* influences and substances, physical body structures and mental–emotional life.

The meaning of 'the heart ruler governing *shén* brightness' in the *Inner Canon* has three interlocking parts. First, the heart is the host of the *shén*: the term heart-*shén* (心神 *xīn shén*) refers to this meaning. Second, the abundance of prenatal and postnatal essences forms the sea of marrow, the brain: the brain and *jīng*-essences are the material basis of *shén míng*. Third, the heart-*shén* must cultivate *míng* brightness and clarity. This part includes the heart-*shén* as ruler of the body form and its visceral systems.

We devote the last part of this chapter to the heart-*shén* without brightness and clarity. The heart without *shén míng* gives rise to disorderly, dimmed, irrational and confused sensory perceptions and emotional responses, mental–emotional instability and poor adaptive ability. The contrast with mental–emotional development and the cultivation of the heart-*shén* highlights the social and health consequences for human mentality without *shén* brightness. The heart-*shén* without brightness causes abnormal, unhealthy *qì* activities, personality problems and a state of mental–emotional disarray.

---

116 《素问·灵兰秘典论篇》: 心为君主之官。神明出焉。… 主明则下安。主不明则十二官危。*Sù wèn, Líng lán mì diǎn lùn piān: 'Xīn wèi jūn zhǔ zhī guān. Shén míng chū yān… Zhǔ míng zé xià ān. Zhǔ bù míng zé shí'èr guān wēi'*

心主神明 The heart-ruler with *shén míng*

The role of the heart as sovereign ruler is to emanate its directing influences (神 *shén*) and clear insight (明 *míng*) (Porkert 1979). The analogy invites us to consider Chinese medicine psychology in terms of two basic ideas: one is the 'heart–ruler with *shén* brightness,' and the other is its opposite, the 'heart–ruler without brightness.'[117] To distil the complexity of psychological phenomena, Chinese medicine emphasizes these two characteristics: the heart-*shén* with and without clear insight. Here is more of the *Elementary Questions* Treatise 8:

> Hence, if the ruler is enlightened, his subjects are peaceful and safe. To nourish one's life on the basis of this results in longevity. There will be no risk of failure till the end of all generations. Thereby ruling the world will result in a most obvious success. If the ruler governs with *shén* brightness, the country is great and glorious.If the ruler is not enlightened, then the twelve officials are in danger. The *shén* pathways are obstructed and impassable.[118] The physical appearance suffers severe harm. To nourish life on the basis of this is disastrous. If ruling without *shén míng*, the country will be ruined. Beware, beware!

The heart-*shén* with brightness enables a normal healthy life, ordering and enlightening the *qì* influences that extend to the mind and personality. To manage its administrative offices, the heart-*shén* receives and coordinates all *zàng shén* cognitive activities and sensory perceptions. To effectively govern, the heart-*shén* must have brightness and clarity. A nation's ruler in fact needs exceptional qualities (明君 *míng jūn*) to govern the country well and bring prosperity to its people. Just as the ruler with *míng* brightness brings great glory to the country, the heart governing with brightness brings a cultured life with rational intelligence and longevity.

　　主 *Zhǔ* means 'to govern' and 'to host.' Just as a country's head of state receives their important guests, the heart host provides lodging for the *shén* and cultivates *míng* brightness. To perform these functions, the ruler of a country and the heart/mind must be bright and rational rather than dull and irrational. If the heart host receives *míng* brightness, the

---

117 心主神明 *xīn zhǔ shén míng*, and 心主不明 *xīn zhǔ bù míng*

118 使道闭塞而不通 *Shǐ dào bì sè ér bù tōng* (使道 *Shǐ dào* means the pathways of the *shén qì* coming and going from the interior to the exterior. For example, when we want to see, the *shén* must go to the eyes; when we want to hear, the *shén* must go to the ears)

nation's people communicate harmoniously through all their agencies and officials. If the heart-ruler cultivates *shén míng*, the effects of virtuous leadership spread throughout the empire. If the heart host is without brightness, then intelligence, cultured life and general health are endangered.

As well as the heart's overall governance of the *zàng fǔ* visceral systems, each of the *zàng fǔ* has their own administrative responsibilities (主 *zhǔ*). The five *zàng* transform and store essential *qì* substances and follow five-phase associations. For example, the heart governs the blood, the vessels and speech, and manifests in the complexion and demeanor; the liver governs vision and manifests in the sinews and nails. The idea of *zhǔ* governance binds together the body and mind, their structures and sensory offices, their mental–emotional activities and responses.

Even before the compilation of the *Inner Canon*, the *Spring and Autumn Annals* (770–404 BCE) warned that the sensory officials, the ears, eyes, nose and mouth, should guard against excess pleasures that could enter and corrupt one's person. If one's mind (心) were 'fixed on an external desire, it could find itself permanently exiled from its welling place' (Yates 1994). Mèng Zǐ (*c.* 372–289 BCE) and Xún Zǐ (330–227 BCE) agreed that although the senses are ruled by the heart/mind, they can interfere with ordering the person. Xún Zǐ explained that the 'sense appetites react mechanically to attractive objects, which cover (蔽 *bì*), blind or obsess them.' But just as importantly, the heart/mind itself can be 'obsessed, so that it blindly pursues a wrong course thinking it to be right' (Nivison 1999, p.792).

If the ruler is not enlightened, disordered sensory perceptions confuse and distort our lived experiences and cause negative emotional responses. Because mental–emotional responses influence the *zàng fǔ* visceral systems and their *qì* functions, disordered responses lead to the situation described in Treatise 8 where, 'If the ruler does not have *shén míng* then the twelve officials are in danger, the *shén* pathways are obstructed, and the physical body is severely damaged.'

府精神明 **The brain essence and** *shén míng*

When the kidney essence forms the bones and marrow, an abundance of the essence is what forms the brain. The *Inner Canon* says the 'brain-essence [is the basis of] *shén míng*,'[119] and here, the 府 *fǔ* or 'palace' is referring to the brain, the sea of marrow. Treatise 17 in the *Elementary Questions*[120] says, 'The five *zàng* provide nourishment and strength to the body. The head is the palace of essence brightness (精明 *jīng míng*).' In commenting on this, Wáng Bīng observes that when the *zàng* are peaceful, the *shén* is protected; and when the *shén* is protected, the body is strong. Then the essence gathers in the head, the 'palace,' producing the brain: this is the material basis of *shén* brightness and intelligence.

The kidney-lifegate stores the inherited and acquired essence, and the abundance of these essences forms the brain. Postnatally, the stomach, spleen and liver *qì* activities produce food essence from our diet, and the lung absorbs clear *qì* essence from the air we breathe. Clear *qì* essence is distilled from the air when we absorb oxygen, while food essence becomes the basis of blood and *qì*. The acquired essences from digestion and respiration, the essential food *qì* and clear air *qì*, nourish and protect both the kidney essence and the brain. The *Elementary Questions* Treatise 21 explains (we have numbered the phrases of this excerpt to facilitate our discussion following):

(1) The *qì* of food enters the stomach, [the stomach] spreads food essence to the liver, and [surplus then flows] into the sinews.

(2) The *qì* of food enters the stomach, the turbid *qì* [the thick food essence] turns to the heart, and [surplus then flows] into the vessels.

(3) The vessel *qì* flows through the channels, the channel *qì* turns to the lung, the one hundred vessels converge in the lung, they transport essence to the skin and soft body hair.

(4) The soft hair [that receives clear *qì*/oxygen from the lung] and fine vessels [that receive food essence from the blood] unite the essence, and they move it to the *fǔ*-palace [where it accumulates]; when the palace is filled with essence there is *shén míng*, it flows to the four *yīn*

---

119 府精神明 *fǔ jīng shén míng*

120 《素问 · 脉要精微论篇》 *Sù wèn, Mài yào jīng wēi lùn piān* ('On the Essential and Finely Discernible Aspects of the Pulse')

viscera, and the body is balanced. We can feel the *qì* at the inch opening [radial pulse], to decide about death or survival.[121]

The passage begins with eating, continues with the formation and distribution of essence, and ends with life and death. 浊 *Zhuó* means the thick and substantial aspects of food *qì* and the 'surplus' used for nourishment. The rich part of food essence goes to form blood, which is then distributed around the body by the heart and the vessels.

While poor nourishment can clearly weaken the brain essence, many diseases in the West are the result of over-consumption of rich foods. Over-consumption disrupts the transformations that begin with food entering the stomach (1). Over-eating injures the middle *qì*, the stomach and spleen cannot transform too much rich, heavy and oily food into essence *qì*, and in any case, our body tissues cannot use it all. Instead of producing nourishing food essence, this kind of diet creates turbid phlegm dampness, a pathological product. Turbidity accumulates in the liver, sinews and flesh, resulting in health problems such as fatty liver and obesity. Furthermore, in the second part (2), the over-consumption of these foods produces so much turbidity the heart cannot use it, and it spreads into the vessels causing hyperlipidemia, atherosclerosis and coronary heart disease.

In the third and fourth parts (3 and 4), the vessels hold the essence from food, and the lung, skin and body hair absorb clear *qì* (oxygen) from the air. The channels and vessels (经脉 *jīng mài*) all converge in the upper *jiāo* and the lung where the clear *qì* and food essences unite. 朝 *Cháo* is an early morning government meeting held at the royal court, and alludes to the lung as the 'prime minister' who distributes orders. The lung's orders, rhythms and *qì* influences, including these united essences, flow through all the vessels and channels and throughout the body, so that when the essence is abundant it fills the head and brain,

---

121 《素问 · 经脉别论篇》: *Sù wèn, Jīng mài bié lùn piān:*

(1) 食气入胃, 散精于肝, 淫气于筋; *Shí qì rù wèi, sàn jīng yú gān, yín qì yú jīn.*

(2) 食气入胃, 浊气归心, 淫精于脉。 *Shí qì rù wèi, zhuó qì guī xīn, yín jīng yú mài.*

(3) 脉气流经, 经气归于肺, 肺朝百脉, 输精于皮毛; *Mài qì liú jīng, jīng qì guī yú fèi, fèi cháo bǎi mài, shū jīng yú pí máo.*

(4) 毛脉合精, 行气于府; 府精神明, 流于四藏, 气归于权衡; 权衡以平, 气口成寸, 以决死生。 *Máo mài hé jīng, xíng qì yú fǔ; **fǔ jīng shén míng**, liú yú sì zàng, qì guī yú quán héng; quán héng yǐ píng, qì kǒu chéng cùn, yǐ jué sǐ shēng.*

the palace of essence (府精 *fǔ jīng*) where the initiating *shén* resides. The brain filled with pure essences forms the material basis for *shén míng* and healthy mentality.

Treatise 17 notes that when *shén míng* is disordered, the patient cannot tie their clothes and they tend to use bad language. Furthermore, if the 'palace of essence' is not filled, *shén míng* is not even possible. Then, the patient's 'head is bent, the eyes are sunken and dull, and the *jīng–shén* are about to be lost.' We can see how cases of depleted essence can present with memory loss, dementia and Alzheimer's disease.

心主修明 The heart-ruler cultivating *míng* brightness

It is the responsibility of the heart-*shén* to cultivate brightness and a healthy inner life.[122] The development of our nature and character are strongly influenced by our family and home environment, our cultural, social and economic background, and the level and style of education we receive. The training and maturity of intelligence (理智 *lǐ zhì*), rationality (理性 *lǐ xìng*) and brightness rely on the correct course of development. So, what is 'correct' for the development of intelligence and healthy psychology?

In Chinese medicine, the notion of 'correct' links the cultivation of social and personal ethical conduct with the familiar concepts of 'correct *qì*' (正气 *zhèng qì*), and its opposite, 'evil *qì*' (邪气 *xié qì*). When *xié*-evil is translated as 'pathogen/ic' in contemporary texts, this more biomedical interpretation helps avoid the moralistic connotations Westerners bring to the idea of 'evil.' Yet Chinese medicine purposely borrowed 'correct' and 'evil' from socio-cultural and administrative ethics to invoke the moral dimensions of social relations. In terms of our intentions and behaviors, the meaning of 'correct' in Chinese culture and medicine takes account of a person's social responsibilities and effectiveness. This is quite unlike the Western preoccupation with personal internal struggles and individual agency. The *Inner Canon*'s political state analogy becomes less metaphoric and more meaningful for the embodied self when we keep both levels of lived experience, the social and personal, in mind.

---

122 心主修明 *Xīn zhǔ xiū míng*

Ethical conduct and the cultivation of virtue have been major topics of Chinese philosophy since very early times. The *Book of Changes*[123] (from *c.* 700 BCE) and the early Daoist and Confucian classics all contain guidance for self-discipline and the cultivation of moral development. Confucianism urges everyone to become a 'true gentleman' (真君子 *zhēn jūn zǐ*), a wise, ethical, exemplary person, and to cultivate strength, respect and wisdom. To cultivate the goodness of human nature, Mèng Zǐ emphasized four virtues: benevolence, dutifulness, propriety and moral intelligence.[124] He stressed that our *qì* (our moral and physical energy) should not be forced but gently lead by the mind (志 *zhì*) that resides with the kidney essence. Confucian practices to cultivate ethical conduct included rituals that helped bind their participants to upright behaviors.

Meanwhile, Daoism advocated quietude and simplicity. Rather than a Confucian and conformist approach, it preferred an attitude that did not seek to control 'spontaneous expression' (无为 *wú wéi*). Daoism links Buddhism's five precepts (against killing, stealing, sexual misconduct, lying, intoxication) with the five virtues (benevolence, wisdom, righteousness, propriety, faithfulness), the five transformative phases (五行 *wǔ xíng*) and the five *zàng* visceral systems.

Buddhism in particular explains how our psychology is shaped by our inherited and acquired influences. In Buddhism, our inherited factors extend beyond our immediate parents, and in this life, acquired influences are gradually formed and developed by study and cultivation. Even though inherited factors shape our innate disposition (such as extroverted/introverted, gentle/rough), qualities such as prudence, patience and stability can be cultivated with 'practice and habit' (新熏 *xīn xūn*).

Chinese Buddhists developed a simple operational definition of psychological health and its cultivation. They identified wholesome and unwholesome mental factors, their resultant mental states, and appropriate corrective strategies. For example, ignorance and mental cloudiness led to misperceptions and confusion and could be corrected by cultivating mental clarity. Aversion and ill-will could be countered by loving kindness, selfish attachment by equanimity, laziness by effort and enthusiasm and so on.

---

123 《易经》 *Yì Jīng*
124 仁义礼智 *rén yì lǐ zhì*

With positive influences and self-cultivation practices, our *shén zhì* resources and activities are potentially 'divine' and 'miraculous' (灵 *líng*). 灵 *Líng* means 'god-like intelligence, flexibility, speed and accomplishment,' such as in the expressions, 心灵 *xīn líng*, 神灵 *shén líng* and 灵魂 *líng hún*. *Líng* denotes a higher level of accomplishment that can occur when we use our *shén zhì* mind in a positive way. Attaining knowledge, fame and material wealth are mundane pursuits, but when we turn our attention to cultivating the Dao and our Buddha-nature, 灵 *líng* arises. This is the attainment of wisdom.

修心明神 *Self-cultivation*

China has a long history of 'cultivating life' (养生 *yǎng shēng*), and there are many topics and practices to guide appropriate diet, exercise, education and sleeping habits. Buddhist, Daoist and Confucian texts recognized that the initiating and acquired *shén* could communicate with each other, and that communication between them would make it possible to stimulate and cultivate one's life potentials. The main purpose of self-cultivation practices therefore, was to encourage their interaction, and by cultivating positive attributes and not cultivating negative ones, we could improve and refine our person.

The *Inner Canon* says we must cultivate our *shén* to ensure it does not scatter or leave the body. When we guard and keep the *shén* with the body, only then is it possible to cultivate life, preserve the true *qì* and attain perfection. For Chinese medicine, cultivating life means harmonizing the 藏神 *zàng shén*. When peaceful and harmonized, *zàng shén* relationships and activities are able to maintain the orderly movement and transformation of our *qì* influences and substances.

Early Chinese thinkers believed that the initiating *shén*, the essence of awareness, loves stillness, whereas the acquired *shén* loves movement and is less stable than the initiating *shén*. The acquired *shén*'s conscious awareness managing the information and sensations of our everyday life is easily influenced by the outside world. But when clear and quiet, the acquired *shén* functions efficiently in the world, its intellect operates smoothly and according to the situation. Chinese thinkers believed that practices cultivating stillness could maintain the acquired *shén*'s connectedness with the deeper, spontaneous knowledge of the initiating *shén*. This is the very basis and importance of self-cultivation.

The *Elementary Questions* Treatise 72 ('Treatise on Acupuncture Methods') is one of the Song dynasty additions to the *Inner Canon*. In a section at the end it explains the importance of returning to the root for self-cultivation:

> Therefore, to cultivate the *shén* correctly, one must always abide with the *dao*, supplement the *shén*, strengthen the root, keep the essence *qì* from scattering and keep the *shén* as one with the body, regardless. If the *shén* stays and is kept whole, it is possible to be true; [but] if human life (人神) is let go, one cannot achieve enlightenment. The importance of true enlightenment is the heavenly mystery, [when] the *shén* guards the heavenly breath, one can re-enter the primary root, this is named the return to the origin.[125]

In this passage, 'heavenly mystery' (天玄 *tiān xuán*) is an expression meaning 'the life essence from heaven/nature.' 玄 *Xuán*, 'the mysterious and unfathomable,' is the black color of the water phase, and the kidney guarding the life essence. 'Heavenly breath' (天息 *tiān xī*) is the foetal respiration (胎息 *tāi xī*) of gestation, when the foetus has only the primary consciousness of the initiating *shén*. 'Return to the origin' (归宗 *guī zōng*) means we return to our earliest beginnings, our ancestors and original roots, and the ideal state of the primordial *qì*. Practices that cultivate 'foetal breath' therefore assist our connectedness with our root origin: and therein lies the key to perfection.

In this way, self-cultivation practices that foster stillness and mindfulness cultivate and harmonize our innate abilities and conscious awareness. The interaction of the initiating and acquired *shén* was thought to be able to repair, correct and brighten the heart (修心 *xiū xīn*); and with heart brightness (明心 *míng xīn*) we would be able to see and cultivate our true nature (性 *xìng*). Self-cultivation practices could sometimes extend to sleeping practices because the acquired and initiating *shén* were thought to be able to harmonize with each other when we are asleep and dreaming. In China, self-cultivation put into practice the belief that

---

125 《素问 · 刺法论篇》：故要修养和神也，道贵常存, 补神固根，精气不散，神守不分，然即神守而虽不去，亦能全真，人神不守，非达至真，至真之要，在乎天玄，神守天息，复入本元，命曰归宗。

Sù wèn, Cì fǎ lùn piān: 'Gù yào xiū yáng hé shén yě, dào guì cháng cún, bǔ shén gù gēn, jīng qì bú sàn, shén shǒu bù fēn, rán jí shén shǒu ér suī bù qù, yì néng quán zhēn, rén shén bù shǒu, fēi dá zhì zhēn, zhì zhēn zhī yào, zài hū tiān xuán, shén shǒu tiān xi, fù rù běn yuán, mìng yuē guī zōng'

to cultivate *shén míng* we must enhance our initiating *shén* abilities and harmonize our acquired *shén* activities with them.

In Chinese thinking, religion is a kind of self-cultivation practice that connects us with the power of nature and the ancestral aspects of our *shén*. Historically, the Chinese people embraced the ethical and religious principles of Daoism, Confucianism and Buddhism. All three encouraged the cultivation of kindness and humanity. They developed simple moral guidelines to help avoid harmful acts and guard against unwholesome influences. When the heart-*shén* is 'correct' (正 *zhèng*, in terms of mindfulness), there is brightness and clarity, and in that state, negative ideas cannot form. To correct the heart and brighten the *shén*, one must conquer oneself, know oneself, be content and be strong. Determination applied to continued, focused, ethical practices develops healthy psychological resources and cultivates the body and mind. This is similar to the idea of the heart-*shén* cultivating *míng*-brightness.

The Chinese understood how our moral conduct and motivations influence our *qì*, and consequently our physical and psychological health. Chinese philosophy and medicine explain that bad behavior occurs when there is a lack of control over the senses; that indulging the senses disturbs the five *shén* and causes confusion and irrational thoughts and impulses; and in that state the five *zàng* can no longer function properly. Whether our heart-*shén* is bright or dim is influenced by inherited factors and childhood experiences, and environmental factors will affect us throughout our life in different ways and degrees. Therefore, Chinese medicine and psychological thought pay a good deal of attention to self-cultivation, self-awakening, enlightenment and the development of our heart road.

Generally, a wholesome and positive environment enriches human life, and ideally the cultivation of heart-*shén* brightness should start early. Yet, positive influences can repair and correct unwholesome ideas and habits at any stage in life. Benevolence and kindness can replace harmful perceptions and habits, and change the heart-*shén* from dullness and confusion to brightness and clarity. The more positive our environment and outlook, the more we can cultivate correct recognition and understanding, and the potential for developing clarity, rationality and radiance increases.

As we know, a normal healthy mental–emotional life in childhood does not guarantee a healthy mind in later life, and nor does an unstable early environment lead inevitably to psychological problems.

A person growing up in an unstable, unsafe or unhealthy environment, however, can form dysfunctional mental–emotional patterns and social disposition more easily than one growing up in a stable, safe and positive environment. They grow up with higher levels of anxiety and suspicion because they see more social darkness and are more susceptible to it. From an anxious and suspicious state, we can more easily form distorted or deluded impressions, anxious/depressive responses and dysfunctional personality traits.

Environmental influences are sometimes subtle, ongoing influences, and sometimes they are sudden and severe. Family, friends and educational environments have a deep and lasting impact on the complex factors and processes of psychological development. Schooling and family life generally provide positive influences and environment, but not in every case and not all of the time. Today, for example, there are many influences that encourage the desire for material possessions, fame, wealth, beauty and success. If persistent and persuasive, those influences can perpetuate habits and heighten desires that result in negative psychological states. Over time, this can affect and change the heart-*shén*, and someone who cultivates such desires may risk more seriously damaging behavior such as theft and corruption.

Sensory information informs human consciousness and in Chinese medicine we associate the qualities of *shén* brightness with the clarity of the senses (官 *guān*) and their apertures (窍 *qiào*). The '*shén* aperture'[126] receives information from all the sensory openings so that the heart-*shén* can coordinate, analyze and interpret this information. In that sense, the *shén* aperture includes all the apertures—the eyes, nose, mouth, ears and tongue, the two *yīn* openings in the lower *jiāo* and the sweat pores of the skin. The correct reception and analysis of sensory information relies on the heart-*shén* hosting and governing brightness and clarity. The heart-*shén* with *míng* brightness enables the receptivity, clarity and flexibility of human consciousness.

The person with heart-*shén* brightness has strong mental and emotional stability and stamina, their adaptive abilities and responses to change are positive and appropriate. Their emotions are not easily disturbed or only briefly disturbed, and they are not easily roused to extreme emotional responses. Such a person is less likely to suffer

---

126 神窍 *Shén qiào*, refers mainly to the 'heart aperture' 心窍 *xīn qiào*, and also includes all the sensory apertures

from psychological disturbance. Their clarity and enlightenment can be observed in their appearance, eyes, temperament and conversation.

心主不明 *The heart-ruler without clarity and brightness*

The person whose *shén* is without brightness, reason and clarity has little mental stamina; their emotional stability and adaptive ability are poor, and their psychological responsiveness and regulative ability are reduced. They find it difficult to face, adapt to, or manage social or environmental changes. They cannot deal appropriately with social interactions, or with success, defeat, setbacks or frustrations. When faced with failure, their mental–emotional state is easily disturbed and their reactions are disproportionate because it is difficult for them to regulate their heart state. This can lead to extreme behaviors such as suicide and murder.

心主不明 *Xīn zhǔ bù míng* is an expression referring to the deterioration of rationality and mental capacity. If there is disruption with any aspect or at any stage of the five *zàng shén* activities, this can impair heart-*shén* clarity and intelligence. When the head of state is 'dull and irrational' (不明 *bù míng*) the country is in chaos and its citizens are in danger. In the same way, when our heart-*shén* is without clarity and lucidity, our inner life is in danger and our psychological activities are disordered.

In the *Elementary Questions* Treatise 8, dullness and confusion 'obstruct the *shén*'s coming and going'[127]—meaning its reception and management of sensory information—and so do sensory desires. Sensory desires can fascinate, captivate, enthral and enchant the heart-*shén*. They can distract and disturb our thinking, and lead to unfortunate extremes (Geaney 2002). When the *shén* aperture is compromised or obstructed by dullness, irrationality or fascination, the five senses still receive information but our inner experiences and interpretations of them are distorted and abnormal. In this state, for example, a person can hear but they cannot listen or understand. If the heart aperture is dimmed, the *shén*'s coming and going is interrupted and impeded. The expression is used medically and in common language to indicate that the heart-*shén* is confused, and that the person has lost their bearings (Qu and Garvey 2009b).

---

127 使道不通 *shǐ dào bù tōng*

Many mental–emotional factors can overcome, confuse and bewilder the heart/mind. For example, the expression 'wealth confounds the heart aperture'[128] describes someone who is obsessed by their desire for wealth. They want only affluence and possessions and will attain them by any means. Similarly, when 'money confounds the heart aperture'[129] it means the person's mind is dimmed and filled up with the desire for money. Their mind is so obsessed they will go to extremes such as fraud or theft to acquire it. 迷 *Mí* means 'to be confused and lost,' and 'to be fascinated, obsessed or fixated.' Where there is 心迷 *xīn mí*, the heart is confused and lost.

In some cases, feelings and emotions overfill and obstruct the heart aperture.[130] Lovers' suicide is an example: when emotions are high, insight is clouded and actions are misguided. When someone is obsessed with power[131] they crave leadership and control and become ruthless in their pursuit of an ever-more powerful position. Even beauty can dim the heart aperture.[132] An example could be the person who becomes sexually inappropriate, addicted or aggressive because they continually lust after younger and more beautiful sexual partners. If their heart-*shén* is fascinated, fixated and obstructed, they will experience this kind of sexual dysfunction; if clear and bright, their sexual behavior is appropriate.

Medically, the terminology for this kind of *shén* disorder is 'phlegm misting the heart aperture.'[133] Sometimes this is given as 'phlegm clouding the heart aperture.'[134] The other common pattern is 'static blood confounds the heart aperture.'[135] Phlegm and static blood are pathological products that cover, obscure or obstruct the apertures, and distort sensory information and heart-*shén* analysis. Their obstruction of our sensory apertures can lead to additional clinical manifestations such as blurred vision, diminished hearing and smell, confusion, hallucinations, delirium, inappropriate or slurred speech or aphasia.

In the context of mental–emotional disorders, pathological products often result from or complicate liver *qì* constraint illness patterns.

---

128 财迷心窍 *cái mí xīn qiào*
129 钱迷心窍 *qián mí xīn qiào*
130 情迷心窍 *qíng mí xīn qiào*
131 权迷心窍 *quán mí xīn qiào*
132 色迷心窍 *sè mí xīn qiào*
133 痰迷心窍 *tán mí xīn qiào*
134 痰蒙心窍 *tán méng xīn qiào*
135 瘀阻心窍 *yū zǔ xīn qiào*

Qì constraint can turn to heat; it can lead to or exacerbate static blood, or the accumulation of untransformed fluids; all of which can dim and obstruct the heart-*shén* aperture. All three—*qì* constraint (with or without fire), static blood, phlegm dampness—are common in cases of depression, mania, insomnia, dementia and psychosis.

Cultivating *shén míng* can prevent negative mental–emotional tendencies disrupting heart-*shén* activities and responsibilities. It is worth remembering, however, that sensory aperture and *shén* pathway obstructions are not only acquired and cultivated over time. They may be inherited, and they can be induced by trauma. Whatever the causative circumstances, and according to Chinese medical methods, treatment follows the pattern/s identified.

For example, in older patients with senile dementia or children with attention deficit hyperactivity disorder (ADHD), a variety of patterns can be found, including phlegm and/or blood stasis obstructing the apertures. Patterns of blood stasis obstructing the apertures in children may have their origins in a history of birth injury. In older people, a history of transient ischemic attacks, silent cerebral infarcts or simple lack of mobility will impair the movement of blood. Phlegm-clearing and stasis-removing medicinals can de-obstruct the channels and apertures, break blood stasis and resolve phlegm dampness. For instance, modifications of Wáng Qīngrèn's (1768–1831) 'Opening Orifices and Activating Blood Decoction' (*Tōng qiào huó xiě tāng*) may be recommended for ADHD and senile dementia patients (Hou 1996).

We know from the *Elementary Questions* Treatise 8 that a lack of *míng* brightness obstructs not only the apertures, but the *shén* pathways. The *shén*'s 'coming and going' takes place via the pathways of sensation and perception that connect and make sense of our internal and external worlds. The *shén* pathways facilitate the coordinated activities and connections between the five *zàng shén* and their sensory offices, tissues and apertures. They should be clear and unobstructed. According to Treatise 8, when a lack of *míng* brightness causes them to become impassable, all the officials are disordered and in danger.

Under normal circumstances, as human life develops and matures, the *shén* pathways become fully developed and well established, but in some cases the pathways, the relationships and connections between the five *shén*, their sense offices and so on, are not properly connected, coordinated or harmonized. This person's sensory perceptions are indistinct or unintelligible; their reception is unclear or illogical;

memory cannot recall past examples or integrate new information; the heart cannot control or manage sensory and cognitive information, it cannot integrate, organize or complete cognitive processes. Autism may be considered an example of disordered *shén* pathways.

From the point of view of Chinese medicine, it seems that the basic mechanism of autism spectrum disorder (ASD) is that the *shén* pathways[136] do not develop, or are not fully established. Research indicates that early intervention can make a significant difference to the ASD child's development; however, later diagnoses offer poor outcomes and the condition becomes difficult or impossible to treat. Although it may be possible to detect developmental indicators as early as 12 months, clinicians cannot diagnose ASD before a child is two years old. It seems that in cases of severe autism, the *shén* pathways are totally closed and impassable and there is no cure. However, in some autistic children, some pathways may be partially established, and in a few of those cases there may be sufficient focus on some or sometimes very specific sensory/cognitive processes to produce special talents. In a very few cases, these circumstances can produce the savant syndrome, and even genius.

* * *

From earliest times, Chinese medicine's analysis of health and illness included the physical, sensory, emotional, social and cognitive aspects of our lived experience. In every age, East and West, a person's character and morality are shaped by their personal actions, and by the social-political systems and the principles and laws that form the identity of their community and its members. Just as greed and arrogance corrupt good governance, anger and discontent pollute our inner life. Just as the head of state with clarity and intelligence brings peace, safety and glory to the whole country, heart-*shén míng* brings rational clarity and accomplishment to our life experience.

The heart-ruler as the host of *shén míng* is both a description of the healthy mind and the causal influence for its ongoing development. By cultivating *shén míng* we are better able to regulate our mental–emotional receptivity and adaptability, and to respond to life's

---

136 神使之道 *shén shǐ zhī dào* (the passageways for the heart-*shén* coming and going, and for its governance driving and coordinating all five *zàng shén*)

successes and failures reasonably and constructively. The heart-*shén* also guides the formation of positive life values and personal qualities: to cultivate cognitive and emotional intelligence, and acquire psychological resilience the *shén* must have *míng* brightness and rational enlightenment.

The heart-*shén* without *míng* brightness is dull and confused, its reception of sensory information is distorted and its interpretations disordered. The accumulation of negative influences on a person's emotions and mentality can lead to body–mind illnesses such as hypertension, asthma or chronic gastritis, or to psychological disorders, psychosis or self-harm. Ethical behavior shapes our mental and emotional life and personality, and the inter-promoting qualities of heart-*shén* brightness, bodily health and a cultured life are said to give longevity. The heart-*shén*'s governance and cultivation of brightness refers to a healthy and positive mental–emotional state.

Míng brightness guides the gradual maturity of our character and humanity. It guides the development of the five *zàng shén* activities from simple to complex, from veiled to unveiled, from dull to clear and bright. Human psychology has great potential and malleability, but the level and degree of clarity and brightness are different for everyone. Although at the beginning of life our acquired *shén* is veiled and dim, positive developmental conditions cultivate the *shén* towards bright, rational intelligence. Over time, as we accumulate positive influences, habits, knowledge and experience, our understanding and recognition gradually improve and the heart-ruler becomes brighter. According to Chinese culture, the heart-*shén*'s clear insight is the light of virtue. When it shines, our eyes are bright and radiate liveliness, and its brilliance and radiance manifests everywhere throughout the empire/body–mind.

Mental health, therefore, is not only a matter for medical research and clinical practice. Every person's psychology is related to inherited factors, shaped by early influences and events, family, personal relationships and the wider socio-cultural environment, and cultivated by personal effort. The heart-*shén* can be influenced and trained throughout life; it can change from dim to bright but also from bright to dim. The accomplishment and maintenance of healthy psychology, and the effective prevention of abnormal psychology, is both a personal and social responsibility.

Chapter 6

Dreams

> The *hún* resides in the eyes during the day and lodges in the liver at night. When it resides in the eyes, it sees; when it lodges in the liver, it dreams. Dreams are the wandering of the *hún*. It traverses the nine heavens and nine earths in an instant.[137]

Dreaming (做梦 *zuò mèng*) is a normal activity during sleep, and scientific research has shown that our attention, learning and re-membering abilities are fundamentally affected by our quality of sleep. Research has also shown that dreams are not meaningless or random images and memory replays. In fact, they appear to be a process of combining, re-evaluating and reorganizing decades of information and memories. Research suggests that this is more than just memory consolidation. While sleeping and dreaming we are synthesizing and learning from the past, discovering rules and relationships, and building mental models imagining or anticipating the future.

According to Chinese medicine, regular sleeping rhythms and dream processes allow the acquired *shén*, five *zàng shén* and initiating *shén* to communicate and harmonize with each other every night while we sleep. While it is possible to enhance our initiating *shén* abilities and to harmonize our acquired *shén* activities with them by applying conscious (acquired *shén*) self-cultivation practices, the dream state is more powerful for their harmonization than the waking state. When we are awake, all our senses are open, receiving and responding to stimulation, information and impressions. When asleep and during the dream state, conscious hearing, seeing, touch, taste and smell are

---

137 From *The Secret of the Golden Flower*, Chapter 2

muted and still. In the absence of sensory distractions, the mind can be focused, the effects of dreams can be stronger and they can leave a deeper impression.

All aspects of the inherited and acquired *shén* are involved in our sleeping and dreaming, not only the *hún*. Of the five *zàng shén*, the *shén*, *hún* and *pò* are especially important. So long as the heart is calm, the *shén* is clear and bright. So long as the *hún* follows the *shén*, we can move skillfully in our outer world and roam freely in our inner world of thought, imagination and sensation.

Visionary states were associated with the *hún*, and according to Zhāng Jièbīn (1563–1640), dreaming, sleeping, floating, absentmindedness and daydreaming all belong to the *hún*.[138] China's largest surviving dream compendium, *An Explication of the Profundities in the Forest of Dreams*,[139] is also from the late Ming dynasty. Hé Dòngrú,[140] its main compiler, catalogued almost five thousand dream examples from the dynastic histories and claimed to have incorporated sections of text by Gé Hóng.[141]

From the *Forest of Dreams*, it is clear that the Chinese thought of dreams as a way for spirits and gods to communicate with them. Dreams could connect one's inner and outer worlds. They could reveal the hidden connections between the future and past, near and distant, imaginary and real, health and illness. Nightmares were sometimes thought to indicate one's personal failings, or to convey appeals from the spirits 'to improve, or suffer the consequences.' The *Forest of Dreams* urges nightmare sufferers to 'undertake a path of critical self-reflection and examination' (Vance 2014). In cases where dreams and nightmares indicated a person's moral corruption, the solution was to cultivate virtue and to reshape their moral fiber based on the messages from their dreams.

The *Forest of Dreams* contains general advice to promote peaceful sleep, similar to that found in late Ming longevity and self-cultivation manuals. General advice related to everyday life, daily routine and diet, and included suggestions to avoid harmful excesses. To cultivate healthy sleeping habits, the *Forest of Dreams* stresses the importance of body position, pillow placement, and the position and height of

---

138 In the *Classified Canon* (1624)
139 梦林玄解 *Mèng lín xuán jiě* (1636)
140 何栋如 Hé Dòngrú (1527–1637)
141 葛洪 Gé Hóng (284–364), Daoist alchemist, medical expert and scholar

the bed. To prevent dreams, nightmares and other sleep disturbances it recommends gymnastics (导引 *dǎo yǐn*), breathing exercises (吐故呐新 *tǔ gù nà xīn*), abstention from grains (却谷 *què gǔ*), talisman water (符水 *fú shuǐ*), sexual practices (房中术 *fáng zhōng shù*), clenching the fists (握固 *wò gù*) and clapping the teeth (叩齿 *kòu chǐ*) (Vance 2014).

做梦机理 The mechanisms of dreaming

Chinese culture and medicine equated good health with virtue and decency, and dreams were regarded as a barometer of health. TCM considers dreams a product of many conscious (acquired) and unconscious (innate) influences. Acquired *shén* dream content consists of day-to-day experiences. Initiating *shén* dream influences include deeper, less immediate content, instinctive urges and preferences and may even contain elements of presage.

Our life experiences are important for dreaming because most dreams are a continuation of day-to-day life. We can observe that they seem to process both recent and distant experiences and memories, as well as difficult incidents and stresses. When we experience conflict, mental–emotional stress or other kinds of problems, these are likely to appear in our dreams at night, and so dreaming is partly a kind of non-conscious *shén* release. Understanding the mechanisms of dreaming, such as the importance of daytime experiences for dreaming, encourages us to unify our self-cultivation practices with our nighttime dreaming and processing.

Normal dreaming, the normal night wandering of the *hún*, does not disturb regular sleeping patterns and is not necessarily remembered in the morning. Excess dreaming is a level of pleasant or unpleasant dreaming that causes restlessness or wakes the sleeper. Excess roaming and frenetic wandering of the *hún* at night in our dreams is the main cause. Excess dreaming includes recurring dreams or waking with a disagreeable feeling or mood, or more seriously, sleepwalking and nightmares.

According to TCM, sleeping and dreaming are important indicators of our physical, spiritual, mental and emotional state, and reveal their connections and conditions. In doing so, dreams can indicate potential and actual disruption and illness. Because dreaming is another kind of *shén zhì* function—one that deals with inner body–mind processes—it reveals the state of our inner life, in particular the state of the *zàng* visceral systems, their *shén* activities and *zàng shén* disorders.

内经 The *Inner Canon*

According to TCM's visceral manifestations theory, the *zàng fǔ* each have their own associations regarding colors, sounds, seasons, animals and so on. Dream content featuring five-phase correspondences, sometimes as unexpected or fantastic combinations of phenomena and images, can signpost which of the five *zàng shén* are disordered.

The *Inner Canon* contains many references to dreams, and two treatises in particular discuss their causal conditions: the *Divine Pivot* Treatise 43,[142] and the *Elementary Questions* Treatise 80.[143] These record a variety of factors that disrupt *qì* movement[144] and cause dreaming and disturbed sleep. For example, in the *Divine Pivot*, lung *qì* repletion causes dreams of fear, sobbing and lifting into the air; and lung-reverting *qì* causes dreams of flying or of queer metal objects. In the *Elementary Questions*, lung *qì* depletions cause dreams of white items, of weapons and combat, or of seeing people executed with their blood flowing in all directions.

The *Divine Pivot* pays more attention to repletion patterns as causative factors, and the *Elementary Questions* to vacuity patterns. The reversal of orderly *qì* movement from both repletion and vacuity patterns disturb *zàng fǔ* functions and cause strange dreams. In extreme cases, this can lead to hallucinations, but in general, dream experiences that disturb sleep are common clinical symptoms signaling mental–emotional disorder. Specific dream content, such as the examples given in the *Inner Canon*, can help identify more specific causal mechanisms or exacerbating pathogenic conditions in all forms of *shén zhì* disease. Table 6.1 summarizes the categories mentioned in the *Elementary Questions* (Treatises 17 and 80) and the *Divine Pivot* (Treatise 43).

Table 6.1: Dreams and disorder in the *Inner Canon*

Disorder	Dreams of ...
Repletion	giving things away
Depletion	receiving things

---

142 《灵枢·淫邪发梦》 *Yín xié fā mèng* ('Excess Evils Release Dreams')

143 《素问·方盛衰论篇》 *Fāng sheng shuāi lùn piān* ('Discourse on Comparing Abundance and Weakness')

144 In the *Inner Canon*, the disruption is often called 厥气 *jué qì* ('reverting *qì*'), a kind of reversal or disturbance of normal *qì* movement

Yīn	(repletion): floods and fear, wading through water (depletion): crossing the sea and feeling scared
Yáng	(repletion): burning, big fires
Yīn and *yáng*	(repletion): killing, harming and destruction
Lung *qì*	(repletion): fear, weeping and sobbing, lifting into the air (*jué qì*): flying, or queer metal objects (depletion): flying, white items, objects made of metal, weapons and combat, seeing people executed, with their blood flowing in all directions
Kidney *qì*	(repletion): being bisected at the waist so that the two parts of the body are separated (*jué qì*): overlooking an abyss, or drowning in water (depletion): boats, shipwrecks and drowning, lying in water, as if there was something to be feared
Liver *qì*	(repletion): being angry (*jué qì*): forests and woods (depletion): fragrant plants and mushrooms, fresh herbs, lying under a tree and does not dare to get up, forests on mountains
Heart *qì*	(repletion): laughing, hilarious or frightening events (*jué qì*): smouldering fire over the hills (depletion): mountains, volcanic eruptions, burning, fires and smoke, stopping a fire, *yáng* items such as dragons
Spleen *qì*	(repletion): joyful singing, feeling so heavy the body is hard to lift (*jué qì*): undulating hills and immense marshes, or storms demolishing buildings (depletion): being hungry, insufficient drinking and eating, putting up walls and building a house, abysses in mountains and marshes
Bladder	(*jué qì*): wandering about (depletion): voyages
Stomach	(*jué qì*): forging and bingeing (depletion): having a large meal
Small intestine	(*jué qì*): communities and thoroughfares (depletion): large cities
Large intestine	(*jué qì*): incontinence (depletion): open fields
Gallbladder	(*jué qì*): litigation and self-mutilation (depletion): fights, trials, suicide
Lower *jiāo*	(repletion): falling (depletion): flying
Genitals	(*jué qì*): sexual intercourse

cont.

Disorder	Dreams of ...
Roundworms	(*jué qì*): crowds, flocking together
Tapeworms	(*jué qì*): attack, destruction, fighting, striking others and inflicting wounds
Neck	(*jué qì*): being decapitated
Legs	(*jué qì*): failing to step forward, living in underground caves or deep in private gardens
Arms and thighs	(*jué qì*): bowing deeply and ceremoniously

While the *Inner Canon* records numerous pathogenic states that can disturb sleep and cause excess dreaming, TCM emphasizes the role of pathogenic heat in agitating the *shén–hún*. Common repletion patterns include heart fire, phlegm fire harassing the heart, and phlegm fire in the stomach. These may accompany or complicate liver *qì* constraint due to mental–emotional stress, and liver *qì* constraint itself can transform into liver fire. *Yīn*-blood depletion patterns can cause empty heat to disturb the *shén* and *hún*. More on this when we discuss insomnia in Part 2.

Chapter 7

Chinese and Western Psychologies

In China and the West today, psychology is a large and growing field of clinical, scientific and cross-disciplinary practice and research. In its first one hundred years, Western psychology focused on the study of individuals, their current situations, their formative life experiences and environment. TCM psychology today also tends to concentrate on the features of the conscious mind, a perspective that focuses on individuals, a single generation, or only a few generations. In both cases, there is a tendency to overlook the chain of human life and its evolution.

In this chapter, we discuss a few aspects of Western and Chinese psychology to help illustrate the application of Chinese medicine for contemporary clinical presentations. We also note some developments in genetics and psychology, and some of Chinese medicine's more recent developments in its approach to psychology. TCM's root-tendency psychology and the tree of human consciousness, for instance, illustrate the root *shén* as the 'root' of the tree and the source of sentient life, an image that recalls the *Divine Pivot*'s Treatise 8, 'The Root *Shén*.'

Comparing the acquired and inherited *shén* with the conscious and unconscious mind

Some recent developments in Western psychology and genetics seem to echo early Chinese conceptions of the ancestral and inherited aspects of *shén*. For example, behavioral genetics and evolutionary psychology are based on the principles of evolutionary biology and natural selection. Epigenetics is the study of heritable genetic changes that are due to environmental and lifestyle factors. Such changes have been observed to persist after cell division and to be passed on to the next generation.

Geneticists have been investigating the inheritance of behavioral traits in humans and other animals since the 1960s. They are looking at the role of evolution and genetics in behavioral traits such as eating, mating, social attitudes and cognitive abilities (Christians and Keightley 2005; Fuller and Thompson 1964). Evolutionary psychologists study the adaptations that have evolved in response to human ancestral environments. They propose that the problems faced by our ancestors produced certain psychological adaptations and argue that many human emotional and cognitive behaviors are generated by evolutionary processes (Cosmides and Tooby 1997; Nairne and Pandeirada 2010).

In Chinese psychological thought, the traces and effects left by 'carved in the bones' experiences affect the individual throughout their own life. Because they are stored deeply within the *shén*, they may also be passed on to the next generation, and can even become part of the collective root *shén* of our ancestors. In terms of their impact on the individual in their own lifetime and perhaps on their descendants' psychological patterns, the 'mechanisms' described by early Chinese psycho-logical thought are similar in some respects to Western psychology's unconscious mind.

From its beginnings in the late 19th and early 20th centuries, Western psychology's notions of the unconscious and conscious mind share some similarities with the prenatal and postnatal aspects of Chinese medicine's *shén*-spirit/mind. The theory of the conscious and unconscious mind was a key feature of psychoanalytic theory, introduced by Austrian psychologists Sigmund Freud (1856–1939) and Josef Breuer (1842–1925). Their theories led to innovative treatment methods for mental illnesses using psychoanalysis. Swiss psychologist Carl Jung (1875–1961), once a close collaborator of Freud, drew on psychoanalytic theory to develop his own ideas about the unconscious mind.

In Western psychology, Jung pioneered dream analysis, founded the practice of analytical psychology and formulated psychological concepts such as 'the archetype' and the 'collective unconscious.'

His version of the theory of the unconscious divided it into two parts: the personal and collective unconscious. The personal unconscious was the same as the Freudian unconscious mind—a reservoir of material that was once conscious but has been forgotten or repressed. Jung's 'collective unconscious' proposed that memory traces from experiences that had been repeated countless times over many generations were collected and distilled, creating a kind of archetypal memory.

Interestingly, the German scholar Richard Wilhelm (1873–1930) had translated *The Secret of the Golden Flower* and sent it to his friend Carl Jung, 'at a time that was critical for my own work' (Jung 1984, originally 1929, p.xiii). Jung found that *The Secret of the Golden Flower* explained two levels of mind in detail: the knowing, conscious awareness and a second level of consciousness. In the English-language version of Wilhelm's translation (1984) these are the 'conscious spirit' (识神 *shí shén*), and the 'primal spirit' (元神 *yuán shén*), respectively. Jung consequently developed a strong interest in East Asian studies such as the *Book of Changes*, Chinese alchemy and Zen Buddhism. In his 1949 Foreword to Wilhelm's translation of the *Book of Changes*, Jung said: 'For more than thirty years I have interested myself in this…method of exploring the unconscious, for it has seemed to me of uncommon significance.'

In Chinese medicine's three aspects of *shén* model, Jung/Wilhelm's 'conscious' and 'primal' spirits are Chinese medicine's 'acquired *shén*' (识神) and 'initiating *shén*' (元神). The knowing conscious awareness of the acquired *shén* (Wilhelm's 'conscious spirit') is very similar to psychoanalytic theory's conscious mind, and there are some parallels between the unconscious mind and early Chinese ideas about the initiating *shén*, Wilhelm's 'primal spirit' (元神 *yuán shén*).

In psychoanalysis, the unconscious is said to deal with dream states, to contain instincts, fears, traumas and passions, and to act like a repository for formative mental–emotional experiences and memories. These memories have a decisive influence on the development and activities of the conscious mind even though they are not normally available to it. To that extent, the unconscious mind shares some similarities with Chinese medicine's prenatal *shén*—the ancestral source of the *shén*, the root *shén* (本神), and its inherited allotment, the initiating *shén*.

Commentators on psychoanalysis's theory of the conscious and unconscious mind sometimes use the iceberg analogy as an image for their apparent and hidden nature. The image of an iceberg divides the mind into observable and submerged realms. The conscious mind is like the small part of the iceberg that is visible above the water's surface; the unconscious mind is like the vast bulk of the iceberg submerged beneath the waterline. We have also previously borrowed the same analogy to help illustrate the inherited and acquired aspects of the *shén*, and their broad similarities with the unconscious and conscious mind (Qu and Garvey 2009a).

In psychoanalytic theory, the unconscious mind is 'submerged' and hidden from conscious awareness. The analogy illustrates Freud's explanation of how our conscious life is driven by forgotten and repressed feelings and memories. The unconscious holds long-forgotten but formative memories and experiences; it contains instincts, traumas and fears, and is closely tied to our dreams. When we apply the analogy to TCM psychology, the 'knowing awareness' of the acquired *shén* is like the part of the iceberg that is visible above the water, and is quite similar to psychoanalytic notions of the conscious mind. In modern Chinese, the word for Western psychology's 'conscious mind' is 意识 *yì shí*.

The Chinese term for the Freudian concept of 'unconscious mind' is 潜意识 *qián yì shí*. The unconscious mind and prenatal *shén* are similar insofar as both are submerged and hidden in nature like the much larger part of the iceberg beneath the waterline. Although the experiences and memories held there are not normally available to our conscious awareness, they have a decisive influence on the development and activities of the conscious mind.

One point of difference between the unconscious mind and the prenatal aspects of *shén* is that Freud's theory of the unconscious relies to a large extent on the mechanism of psychological repression. So, as well as distant and forgotten memories, the Freudian unconscious contains socially unacceptable ideas, wishes and desires. Importantly for psychoanalysis, the unconscious mind also retains traumatic experiences and painful memories that have been repressed from our conscious awareness.

During the late 1800s, this led Freud and Breuer to identify connections between psychical trauma and neurotic defense. Their treatment of neuroses such as hysteria was based on their thesis that the condition was a result of a psychical trauma that had been repressed and lost to the patient's conscious memory. According to Freud, the repression of the trauma was a defense mechanism, even though the repression itself could cause conflicted and misdirected impulses, obsessions and sleep disturbances (Freud 1977). These days, Western psychology's anxiety, depressive, obsessive, psycho-somatic and mood disorders have replaced neurosis as a disease category. However, there is still some value for us in having a broad understanding of the term 'neurosis' and its contrast to 'psychosis.' The neurotic patient experiences a distorted, dimmed, confused or exaggerated view of reality, whereas the psychotic patient experiences episodes of complete loss of contact with reality, such as delusions and hallucinations.

The plasticity of the psychological model

Each of us has our own unique *shén*, our own unique disposition, talents, traits and mental–emotional patterns. Our individual *shén* patterns are derived from our pre- and postnatal influences and develop according to their interactions and activities. As well as all the possible ancestral and inherited traits passed down to us through many generations, each of us has very different acquired *shén* influences that are formed and cultivated by our life experiences, environments, habits and practices. Thus, even people who live in the same environment and family can develop very differently.

Early Chinese psychological thought recognized how our postnatal environment, as well as our ancestral and inherited resources, influenced our psychological development. As the conscious awareness of feelings, sensations, thoughts and attitudes, the acquired *shén* is bound by habit and the conditioning of our personal, social and cultural history. As the Chinese saying goes: 'Close to cinnabar you are red [loyal and sincere], close to ink you are black [dark].'[145]

A person's psychological traits are largely decided by their initiating *shén* allotment, which is then influenced by their acquired *shén* activities. If the initiating *shén* is positive, their heart-*shén* aperture is open and their *shén* pathways are smooth and unobstructed. Such a person is cultured and adaptable. If their initiating *shén* allotment includes negative traits, their heart-*shén* aperture is not clear and

---

145 近朱者赤，近墨者黑 *Jìn zhū zhě chì, jìn mò zhě hēi*

the *shén qì* pathways are obstructed. They are stubborn, uncultured, irrational and inflexible. It will be difficult for this person to change their personality and for others to influence them.

Recent developments in TCM psychology

The tree of human life and consciousness

Chinese scholars of psychology, such as Professor Sūn Zéxiān (孙泽先 1946–) of the Liaoning University of TCM, use the metaphor of a tree to explain the relationship between the prenatal and postnatal *shén*. As an image of human consciousness, the tree is more appropriate than the iceberg analogy and describes Chinese medical thought more clearly. It conveys ideas about nature and life that are prevalent in traditional Chinese culture. A tree exists harmoniously with its environment: it is one with 'heaven and earth' (天地 *tiān dì*). The image invokes the *Divine Pivot* Treatise 8 (本神 *Běn shén*), and the idea of the root *shén* as the source of sentient life.

The tree is a more profound and complete metaphor for human consciousness because the iceberg is cold, lifeless and floating without root. By contrast, the tree is alive and organic, it is rooted in the earth and its branches grow and spread upwards towards heaven. As a metaphor for human psychology, the tree shows the three aspects or levels, all of which influence and interact with each other. The above-ground part of the tree—the visible part of the trunk, the branches and leaves that extend out into the world—are like the acquired *shén*, the observable level of conscious awareness.

The heartwood within the trunk and the underground root system are like the initiating *shén*. This is a deeper, inner level of instinctual abilities, drives and behaviors, similar in some respects to Western psychology's unconscious mind. Within the core of the root system lie the innate conditions, activities and responses, including the psychological archetypes and natural instincts, that are the fundamental root nature of human mentality. The inner core of the tree's root system is likened to the root *shén*, the deepest level of the unconscious mind that holds psychological archetypes and the root source of human life.

The tree's large, complex root system spreads downward into the soil. This part of our mind connects with the earth, whose influences are needed to support our inner balance and stability. Above the earth, the tree is embraced by heaven. It harmonizes with its surrounding influences—air, sunlight and water—just as the acquired *shén* must harmonize with its surroundings. To understand the objective world, the acquired *shén* perceives and experiences the outside world like the tree growing above the ground. To survive and grow normally, the two parts of the tree above and below the ground need to harmonize with their environments. TCM sees the integration of nature (天 *tiān*) and human beings (人 *rén*) as the harmonization of a deep inner world with its environment and surroundings.

Therefore, in TCM, the notion of psychological 'integration' means more than a person's social and interpersonal connectedness. Like the branches and roots of a tree, the postnatal and prenatal *shén* communicate with, support and influence each other. Their psychological growth and development are opposite and complementary: the acquired *shén* continually explores the outer world like the branches and leaves of a tree that grow upward and outward; the prenatal aspects of *shén* extend deeply into the inner world like the roots of the tree spreading downwards. The former is a process of outward exploration and the latter is a process of introspection and self-examination. The larger, stronger and more stable the tree's root system, the higher the branches grow and the more the leaves flourish.

Root-tendency psychology

The success of the tree metaphor in China today is that it reflects very early as well as recent Chinese psychological thinking. The growth (*yáng* transformations) of above and below ground aspects of human life is complemented by natural processes of return and decay (*yīn* transformations). The tree of human life also captures the content and meaning of Chinese medicine's 'root-tendency psychology,'[146] a branch of TCM psychology developed in recent times through the observations of certain psychological and behavioral phenomena. Its name evokes the Chinese expression: 'a fallen leaf returns to its roots.'[147] The expression in turn echoes the *Classic of the Law and its Power* (*c.* 460 BCE), where it says, 'All living things, return to their roots.'[148]

---

146 归根心理学 *guī gēn xīn lǐ xué*
147 叶落归根 *yè luò guī gēn*
148 《道德经》：夫物芸芸，各归其根。*Dào dé jīng: 'Fū wù yún yún, gè guī qí gēn'*

Though quite common, root-tendency behaviors are not easy to explain. Just as a tree's leaves fall and return to its roots, whales, turtles, fish and birds migrate vast distances to return to their birthplace and according to the life and reproductive cycles of their ancestral and inherited biology. Humans experience the root-tendency phenomena when feeling homesick or wanting to 'find one's roots.' We have all observed how some friends and loved ones feel a strong desire to return to their homeland as they get older.

In China, root tendency is also seen in people's regard for their parents and the respect paid to their elders and ancestors. Root tendency is what drives the biggest migration of people every year during the Spring Festival in China. No matter how far or how difficult the journey, and no matter how busy they are, all Chinese people rush back home from all directions within China and abroad for a reunion with family members. The celebration is especially to pay our respects to our parents because they gave us life and brought us into the world. They are the root of our life.

The root-tendency phenomenon is thought to be the basis of religious beliefs and practices. The Chinese word for 'religion' is 宗教 *zōng jiào*. 教 *Jiào* means mind training, enlightenment and education. 宗 *Zōng* is related to race and culture and means the ancestral and original root (宗根 *zōng gēn*). 宗 *Zōng* is both the origin of an ancestral line and an important gathering of family members and ancestors. The upper part of the character (宀) is a dwelling or roof that covers and contains the lower part (示). 示 *Shì* means to show and display. It is the image of heavenly light radiating from the sun, moon and stars, the ancestor and spirit influences illuminating human life from the heavens (see Bromley *et al.* 2010; Wieger 1965; and the discussion on the character for 神 *shén*, in Chapter 1).

* * *

For effective clinical practice in the area of TCM psychology it is essential to understand the *shén*. In Part 1 we have seen how the *shén* governs our physical appearance and psychological character, and how the term refers to the many abilities of human life that have been developing continuously for millions of years. The three aspects of *shén*—the root, initiating and acquired *shén*—are three levels of mental–emotional resources, character, personality and intelligence that shape our personal traits.

The root *shén* is inherited from our ancestors and is the source of human life in a hidden state before life begins. After birth, it is stored in the lifegate within the kidneys. Just as the source *qì* is the diffuse influence of inherited and constitutional life information, the *shén* that resides in the kidney-lifegate constitutes the ancestral root and source of our mental–emotional life. The root *shén* is the foundation of the initiating *shén* and together they are the inherited, prenatal aspects of *shén*.

The initiating *shén* is the beginning of life. It carries the instinctual responses and activities that pass from one generation to the next. The initiating *shén*'s undifferentiated life power carries the many potentials and abilities of human life and its biological evolution to instigate, develop and continue a new individual life. It carries basic life functions, instinctual and survival activities and drives, and our sensory and language abilities. Although it is without conscious awareness and knowledge, the initiating *shén* is the beginning and foundation of our conscious mind and psychological makeup.

The acquired *shén* is our postnatal conscious awareness. After birth, the acquired, knowing *shén* is produced by the activities of the five *zàng shén* and their sensory offices. The *zàng shén* are the differentiated postnatal aspects of the initiating *shén*. The heart-*shén* governs the reception and analysis of the sensory, emotional and cognitive activities that comprise our stream of conscious awareness, our inner life. The interactions between inherited potentials and acquired resources, the prenatal and postnatal *shén*, have far-reaching implications for every person's psychological and emotional development.

From the point of view of the tree of human life, the root and origin of life are like the tree's heartwood, its extended root system underground and the inner core of the roots. In TCM psychology, evolutionary information stored in the root *shén* enables human life. The initiation of new life begins at conception when the two parental essences combine. This is the initiating *shén*. The ovum and sperm are the new individual's original *yīn* and *yáng* essences, and the prenatal aspects of *shén* are the basis of postnatal human life, its physical form and development.

The conscious knowing of the acquired *shén* is like the branches and leaves that extend out into the world. The acquired *shén* consists of the coordinated analysis of the constant stream of sensory information received by the five *zàng shén*. The heart-*shén*'s powers of perception, understanding, cognition, memory, planning, knowing, analysis, study, language and intelligence are closely tied to our physical resources, *qì* substances and influences.

For Chinese medicine practitioners, an awareness of the three aspects of *shén* can adjust our clinical focus to consider a broader, more generational perspective. Even though it is impossible to conceive the countless formative experiences and memories that contribute to the psychological patterns of every individual, our individual lives are an expression of our origins. The initiating *shén* decides our psychological model or type; its characteristics, and the strong roots of its long history, govern our whole life. Our acquired *shén* activities, environment and other influences can modify them to some degree. We can train and cultivate these tendencies and improve our mental and emotional abilities and patterns with study, effort and perseverance.

Chinese medicine's understanding of the *shén*, including its three aspects and five *zàng shén*, is essential for the diagnosis and treatment of mental–emotional illnesses. In Part 2, we turn to the clinical applications of these ideas in the practice of Chinese medicine psychology.

PART 2

DIAGNOSIS AND TREATMENT

In Part 2, we discuss the clinical manifestations, diagnosis and treatment of common psychological disorders. Our mental–emotional life can be affected by factors from within or outside the body. *Qì* or blood vacuity, *yīn–yáng* imbalance and disturbance due to pathogenic factors (such as heat, dampness, phlegm, static blood, fire toxins) can all disrupt 神志 *shén zhì* activities. When the five *zàng shén* are disordered, the body–mind relationships disintegrate and separate, and this results in various physical, mental and emotional signs and symptoms. In all cases of mental illness (神志病 *shén zhì bìng*) the heart-*shén* can no longer host and govern *shén míng* (神明), the clarity and power of human conscious awareness. When the heart's governance of *shén míng* is disrupted, the *shén* cannot process, coordinate or complete the information transmitted from the senses.

Classic texts and formulas provide accurate information for diagnosis and effective strategies for treatment, and we begin this section with some of these illness categories. Many of Chinese medicine's earliest examples of what today we know as psychological disorders were first recorded by Zhāng Zhòngjǐng (张仲景 150–219 CE). The disorders in his *Essential Prescriptions of the Golden Cabinet* are representative of disharmony, repletion, depletion and constraint patterns that are still common in contemporary clinical practice.

Zhāng Zhòngjǐng's analyses are the basis for later developments in Chinese medicine theory and practice. His *Golden Cabinet* and *Treatise on Cold Damage*[149] texts identify the manifestations of complex illness dynamics, and match them with guiding formulas that concisely target their patho-mechanisms. Zhāng Zhòngjǐng's 'classic formulas' (经方 *jīng fāng*) are famous for their relevance and effectiveness and are widely used in China and the West today.

Practitioners will be aware that many of the formulas discussed here in Chapter 8 are well known for their treatment of psychological disorders, while some can be applied more widely in practice. In Chapter 8, we concentrate on the formulas' relevance for mental–emotional disorders. The conditions listed in bold refer to the illness headings and indications presented throughout the chapter, as a reminder of a formula's flexibility and its potential applications beyond the topic in which it is presented.

TCM applies the theories explained in Part 1 to the analysis of psychological health and illness. Part 2's presentation of early and contemporary illness categories illustrates their application and relevance for healthcare and clinical practice today. The initial topics and early illness categories note the main indications for diagnosis and pattern identification so that practitioners can apply classical Chinese medicine data to modern disease categories and presentations. The discussion of common contemporary illness categories expands on classical strategies and formulas and maps out some of their extended applications.

For the analysis of diagnostic data, we apply *shén zhì* theory to describe the nature of *qì* disturbances causing *shén* consciousness, body–mind–emotion, and cognitive–sensory disorders. The *shén zhì* model encompasses information regarding the patient's inherited attributes and acquired influences, their body–mind and essence-*shén* (精神 *jīng shén*) resources, the interactions between the five *zàng shén* (五藏神) and their associated sensory faculties and visceral systems, including the *zàng fǔ* physiological (*qì*) activities, the *yáng qì*, *yīn*-blood, fluids and essence. For diagnosis, we observe the manifestations of *shén* in our patient's appearance and movements, their way of talking and responding, their facial expression and demeanor, their eyes (眼神 *yǎn shén*) and complexion (神色 *shén sè*).

---

149 《金匮要略》 *Jīn guì yào lüè*, and 《伤寒论》 *Shāng hán lùn* (both originally *c*. 220 CE)

Chinese medicine interprets mental–emotional signs and symptoms as it does any body–mind activity. Rather than treat a physical or psychological disease, the approach is to adjust and harmonize *qì* influences, movements and transformations. To adjust and harmonize the patient's internal environment the TCM clinician must understand and identify complex illness dynamics. With an accurate image of the illness and its patho-mechanisms we can determine appropriate treatment methods and individualize prescriptions.

Appropriate treatments remove pathogenic influences, replenish depleted *qì* substances, restore correct *qì* movements and harmonize *zàng fǔ* functions. Strategies for stagnation and constraint, for example, must 'transform phlegm dampness,' 'dredge the liver' or 'dissolve stagnation and eliminate vexation.' Depleted *qì* substances and visceral systems must be replenished and strengthened. Because our mind, body and emotions are all manifestations of *qì*, the therapeutic adjustment of *qì* adjusts all aspects of the self.

Chapter 8

Illness Categories

There are many kinds of signs and symptoms that signal *shén zhì* disorders. Visual hallucinations indicate liver-*hún* disorder and disharmony between the *shén* (神) and *hún* (魂); paresthesias indicate lung-*pò* disorder and *shén–pò* disharmony; hysterical paralyses signal *hún–pò* (魂魄) disharmony and so on. In some older patients, forgetfulness and memory loss indicate depleted *jīng*-essence.

Age-related cognitive decline illustrates the *jīng–shén* relationship, one of the *qì*-based body–mind relationships described by TCM basic theory. As the kidney *jīng*-essence declines, kidney-*zhì* activities become disordered and their heart-*shén* analysis is no longer supported. With this kind of heart-*shén* and kidney-*zhì* disharmony, solving complex problems and remembering names and appointments, for example, becomes more and more difficult. The classics record many of these physiological relationships and the patho-mechanisms of disorder, and we begin with some of them.

Early illness categories

The disorders and illness categories recorded in the classics are at the heart of many contemporary psychological diseases and clinical presentations. Their identifying features and guiding formulas are applicable to many modern illness categories, such as anxiety and depression, and to psychological disorders associated with menstruation, pregnancy and menopause. Classic formulas can be deployed, modified and reinterpreted according to individual illness patterns, specific patient conditions and the changes in their clinical presentations over time.

Shén–hún disharmony

神魂 *Shén–hún* disharmony occurs when the *shén* and *hún* fail to follow one another. It is mainly caused by mental or emotional stress. Alternate names are '*shén* is gone' (走神 *zǒu shén*) and '*hún* is fallen' (掉魂 *diào hún*). When the harmony of the *shén–hún* relationship is disrupted, the processes involved in perception, cognition, planning, analysis and judgment are interrupted and incomplete. This situation can produce many kinds of signs and symptoms.

Someone with *shén–hún* disharmony will to some extent be inattentive or indifferent to their external environment. Typically, the patient watches but sees nothing. While such behavior can indicate serious mental illness, it is common in a mild form for those of us who easily slip into distracted states such as daydreaming or absent-mindedness. Disturbances to normal sleep patterns, such as insomnia, dream-disturbed sleep and sleepwalking, are another important feature.

An acute or long-term pattern where the *shén* and *hún* fail to follow each other can develop into more serious *shén zhì bìng*, a broad category similar to psychosis. Psychosis is diagnosed in cases of grossly disorganized speech and behavior, auditory, visual, olfactory, gustatory and tactile hallucinations, catatonic stupor or excitement and agitation. From the TCM point of view, the heart-*shén* is severely disordered and unable to govern *shén* brightness. Visual hallucinations, trance, catatonic stupor or hysterical paralysis indicate that the liver-*hún*'s governance of vision, sinews and movement is also disordered. The patient's feelings of physical discomfort are due to the associated body–mind disharmony.

Less severe types of *shén zhì bìng* roughly correspond to modern psychiatry's neurotic, depressive and anxiety disorders. Although there are no physical changes or explanation for many of the less serious *shén zhì* disorders, it is important to remember that symptoms are not feigned and should be distinguished from malingering and factitious behaviors and disorders (Garvey 2001).

Shén–pò disharmony

Some patients with mental illness present with paresthesia. Some cannot feel burning, seem insensitive to cold, or their clothes are inappropriate for the weather. Some psychiatric patients do not realize they smell bad, are dirty, or are eating stool. Others present with abnormal psychomotor activities and mannerisms, such as pacing, rocking, grimacing and posturing, or with more serious repetitive, non-functional motor-behavior, such as head-banging, self-biting or hitting, or picking at their skin or bodily orifices. Even though their skin and nasal tissues are physically normal, the *shén–pò* (神魄) relationship and its transmission and interpretation of sensory perceptions are disordered.

The lung-*pò* participates in the physiological and sensory functions of the skin and nose to receive tactile and olfactory information. A disordered *shén–pò* relationship therefore can be identified in cases presenting with sensory dysfunction affecting smell and touch. The patient's perceptions are lessened, dull, hypersensitive, exaggerated, distorted or unrelated to real conditions.

The features described by Zhāng Zhòngjǐng in the *Essential Prescriptions of the Golden Cabinet*'s **lily bulb disease** are a clear example of the *shén–pò* disharmony. The patient's experience of hot and cold sensations is unrelated to fever, chills or environment; although their food is delicious, they find its smell repugnant; they may want to walk about, but soon become tired. The desire to eat with difficulty swallowing and the need for rest with restlessness is also typical of disharmony between the body and mind. The patient's physical responses are discordant with heart-*shén* inclinations.

It is helpful to keep in mind that Chinese medicine's *shén* disorders are not restricted to Western psychological diseases. For example, *shén–pò* disharmony signs and symptoms such as loss of smell can occur in the early stages of Parkinson's disease and other degenerative neurological disorders. They can occur in patients with diabetes, or 'consumption–thirst disease' (消渴病 *xiāo kě bìng*), an illness category that was recorded in the *Golden Cabinet* (Lines 13–14, see Chapter 4).

Hún–pò wandering

The *Divine Pivot* Treatise 43 divides dream states into three general kinds:

- *yīn–yáng* (water and fire)

- repletion and depletion (flying and falling, full and hungry)

- 魂魄 *hún–pò* wandering.

Hún–pò wandering is a form of *shén–hún* disharmony. Its most common clinical manifestations are vivid, **disturbing dreams** and **sleepwalking**. In the *Divine Pivot*, *hún–pò* wandering is due to *yīn–yáng* imbalance, and the *Golden Cabinet* identifies the role of depleted blood and *qì*:

> [Line 11.12] When evil crying[150] disquiets the *hún* and *pò*, this means that blood and *qì* are scant. Scantiness of blood and *qì* is associated with the heart. The patient experiences fear, desires to sleep, dreams of traveling afar, *jīng shén* are separated and dispersed, the *hún–pò* are wandering abnormally.[151] Debilitation of yin causes insanity-withdrawal (癲 *diān*), debilitation of *yáng* causes mania (狂 *kuáng*).

Depleted blood affects the liver-*hún*, weakened *qì* affects the lung-*pò*, and the heart rules the *qì* blood and the *hún–pò*. When *qì* and blood are depleted, the *shén* is fearful and unsettled, the *jīng*-essence is dissipated, the *hún–pò* relationship is disrupted, causing the patient to wander anxiously, and they experience excess and disturbing dreams. The patient dreams of travelling and, in some cases, this may include episodes of sleepwalking. A worsening of the condition leads to *yīn* and/or *yáng qì* insufficiency and to *diān* withdrawal or *kuáng* mania.

The sleepwalker is able to accomplish complex motor behavior even though they are still asleep. Together, the liver-*hún* and lung-*pò* can manage the functions of vision and movement to the extent that the patient can negotiate obstacles. But the *hún–pò* cannot take the place of the heart-*shén* in engaging conscious awareness, coordinating all five *zàng shén* and governing *shén zhì* activities. Thus, when sleepwalking, the patient has a blank stare, reduced alertness and their responsiveness is diminished.

Normal perception, processing and completion of cognitive information require that the *shén* and *hún* must follow each other, that the heart-*shén* recalls (意 *yì*), and that *yì*-ideation is stored (志 *zhì*). Without the heart-*shén* in charge, the body and mind are not unified. The patient is unresponsive, their movements are abnormal, they cannot remember their sleepwalking and may not know where they are when they awaken out of their bed. It is best not to suddenly wake the sleepwalker in case their *shén* flees.

---

150 邪哭 *xié kū* 'evil crying': emotional disturbance with no apparent reason, as if caused by evil ghosts
151 魂魄妄行 *hún pò wàng xíng*

Shén wandering

Like sleepwalking, *shén* wandering (神遊 *shén yóu*) is another example of the *shén* and *hún* failing to follow each other. The clinical signs and symptoms are similar to *hún–pò* wandering but the disturbance is more serious and instead of occurring at night while asleep, *shén* wandering takes place during the day while awake. *Shén* wandering can be compared to modern psychiatry's **dissociative amnesia**. The patient experiences confusion and inability to recall past memories. They can undertake sudden and unexpected travel away from their home or work with amnesia and identity confusion. They can even assume a new identity. Whether the patient presents with manifestations of *shén* or *hún–pò* wandering, they will be extremely anxious and under great pressure.

Lily bulb disease

In the *Golden Cabinet*, Zhāng Zhòngjǐng's description of 'lily bulb disease,' or 'hundred union disease' (百合病 *bǎi hé bìng*) records the diagnostic features of ***shén–pò* disharmony**:

[Line 3.1] It is said that lily bulb/hundred-union disease is so-called because the hundred vessels share the one origin, which can cause disease everywhere. It manifests in desire to eat but then not being able to, frequent taciturnity, desire to sleep but not being able to, desire to walk but not being able to, desire to eat and drink but finding some foods delicious and with others unable to bear even the smell, signs resembling a cold condition but without cold, signs resembling a heat condition but without heat, bitter taste in the mouth and red urine. None of the various medicines can treat it. Taking medicine results in violent vomiting and diarrhoea, as if the patient were possessed. The physical form seems to be in harmony and the pulse is faint and rapid.

百合 *Bǎi hé* has two meanings. *Bǎi hé* is the word for 'lily bulb,' the main medicinal used to treat lily bulb disease. The other meaning is 'hundred union,' which is the literal translation and the explanation of the mechanism of the disease and its development. As an alternate name for lily bulb disease, 'hundred union disease' alludes to the lily bulb's many converging layers, to the disease's complex manifestations and to its location in the 'hundred vessels.' The hundred vessels have a single origin: the heart governs the blood and vessels, and the lung assembles the hundred vessels. Thus, the hundred union disease involves all the vessels, and this means it can cause disease everywhere. In relation to the heart and lung, the pattern is one of depleted *yīn*-fluids, which deprives the hundred vessels of nourishment.

百合病 *Bǎi hé bìng* is attributed to **heart and lung *yīn* vacuity** with ***shén–pò* disharmony** caused by internal dryness and heat, a condition that will worsen if sweating is induced. *Bǎi hé bìng* can occur due to external or internal factors. Residual heat may linger after an externally contracted febrile disease; or, emotional frustration may give rise to constraint that transforms into pathogenic heat. Both damage the heart and lung *yīn*-fluids. Depleted *yīn*-fluids is a physiological state that is often accompanied by internal empty heat.

For this condition, Zhāng Zhòngjǐng recommends 'Lily Bulb and Anemarrhena Decoction' (百合知母汤 *Bǎi hé zhī mǔ tāng*):

Bǎi hé zhī mǔ tāng (Lily Combination)

Bai he (Bulbus Lilii)   30g

Zhi mu (Rhizoma Anemarrhenae)   30g

The formula nourishes heart and lung *yīn*, clears *yīn* vacuity heat, moistens dryness, and harmonizes the *shén–pò*.

With appropriate clinical presentations (as per the *Golden Cabinet*, Line 3.1), *Bǎi hé zhī mǔ tāng* may apply to patients with irritability, dizziness and disorientation, clinical **depression** and **anxiety** disorders, cough, obsessiveness, **insomnia**, **sleepwalking**, erratic behavior and mood swings, peri-menopausal or **menopausal syndrome**.

Bǎi hé zhī mǔ tāng is selected in cases where upper *jiāo* signs and symptoms (such as thirst, dizziness and insomnia) are pronounced.
Modifications:

- With feverishness and stranguria, – *Zhi mu* and + *Hua shi* = ***Bǎi hé huá shí sàn***

- With cough and restlessness, – *Zhi mu* and + *Sheng di huang* = ***Bǎi hé dì huáng tāng***

A typical feature of lily disease patients is that they present with an unusually wide and puzzling variety of subjective symptoms. The disorder is characterized by mental strain, listlessness, abstraction, sleeplessness and lack of appetite. Emotional lability and depressed mood are often accompanied by unclear and changeable sensations of temperature, feeling both hot and cold. Patients are likely to experience dizziness, confusion and muddled thinking, with poor focus and unclear goals. They are often reluctant to talk; they may have an unpleasant or metallic taste in the mouth, a red tongue, yellow urine and a faint, rapid pulse.

While TCM textbooks recommend Zhāng Zhòngjǐng's lily disease formulas for the treatment of heart and lung *yīn* vacuity patterns, the features described in Line 3.1 clearly indicate the *shén–pò* disharmony.

Plum pit qì

Zhāng Zhòngjǐng did not use the illness name 'plum pit *qì*' (梅核气 *méi hé qì*) in the *Golden Cabinet*. The name was given later because of its principle symptom, the feeling that there is a lump or something lodged in the throat. Chapter 22 'Women's Miscellaneous Diseases,' Line 22.5 describes this as: 'When a woman has a feeling in the throat like a lump of roasted meat.' Zhāng Zhòngjǐng's Pinellia and Magnolia Bark Decoction (半夏厚朴汤 *Bàn xià hòu pǔ tāng*) is the guiding formula.

Bàn xià hòu pǔ tāng
(Pinellia and Magnolia Bark Decoction)

Zhi ban xia (prepared Rhizoma Pinelliae)	12g
Hou po (Cortex Magnoliae Officinalis)	9g
Fu ling (Sclerotium Poriae Cocos)	12g
Sheng jiang (Rhizoma Zingiberis Recens)	15g
Zi su ye (Folium Perillae)	6g

The formula transforms phlegm, dissipates clumps, benefits the stomach and strengthens the spleen. These actions and the ingredients' bitter, acrid, fragrant and warming qualities, effectively release constraint and restore correct movement of *qì*.

With the appropriate clinical manifestations (as in the *Golden Cabinet*, Line 22.5), the formula is recommended for **plum pit** *qì*, sore, parched or itchy throat, **anxiety**, worry, **depression**, **insomnia**, **psychosis**, epilepsy, peri-/**menopausal syndrome**, vomiting, irritable bowel syndrome (IBS), bi-polar disorder.

Modifications:

- Severe anxiety and insomnia, + *Shan zhi zi, Lian qiao, Huang qin*

- Hyperthyroidism, + *Xia ku cao, Bai shao, Xiang fu*

- *Qì* vacuity patterns, + *Ren shen* (or *Dang shen*), *Gan cao*

The sensation of 'plum pit *qì*' or 'plum stone throat' occurs because of emotional factors and is due to **qì constraint and phlegm accumulation** in the throat. A mental–emotional incident or trauma disrupts liver coursing and discharge, and the liver channel travels from the chest area through the neck and behind the throat. The internal (mental–emotional) etiological factors, the subjective feelings of obstruction and their location in the throat indicate that the liver *qì* is not flowing freely. When *qì* constraint disrupts spleen and stomach *qì* transformations, the pattern includes the congealing of phlegm dampness.

Plum pit *qì* is an early example of the 郁证 *yù zhèng* 'constraint pattern' and describes a type of immaterial, 'formless' (无形 *wú xíng*) obstruction: *qì* stagnation with the accumulation of non-substantial phlegm in the liver channel where it passes behind the throat. Biomedical investigations reveal no physical or pathological changes and can find no organic reason for the sensation. Nevertheless, plum stone throat is a real disorder and is very common today. In the West, plum pit *qì* is well known too: *globus hystericus* was once a serious psycho-emotional disease.

In these cases, as well or instead of the sensation of a lump in the throat, there may be difficulty swallowing or loss of voice. Accompanying signs and symptoms can include tightness or fullness in the chest, cough, poor appetite, nausea and vomiting, fainting, headaches and fatigue. The patient may have issues with anxiety or depression. Their symptoms worsen with stress, sadness, anger and frustration.

Visceral agitation

In the *Golden Cabinet*, Zhāng Zhòngjǐng describes the 'visceral agitation' (脏/藏躁 *zàng zào*) illness category using the image of a woman who weeps constantly, 'as if she were haunted.'

[Line 22.6] Woman's visceral agitation manifests in a tendency to sorrow and desire to weep, as if possessed by ghosts, and frequent yawning and stretching. Liquorice, Wheat and Jujube Decoction (甘麦大枣汤 *Gān mài dà zǎo tāng*) governs.

Gān mài dà zǎo tāng
(Liquorice, Wheat and Jujube Decoction)

Gan cao (Radix Glycyrrhizae)	9g
Xiao mai (Fructus Tritici)	15g
Da zao (Fructus Jujubae)	10 pieces

The formula harmonizes the emotions and the *qì* of the five *zàng*; it settles the heart-*shén*, liver-*hún* and lung-*pò*, harmonizes the spleen and stomach *qì* and relaxes tension.

With the appropriate clinical manifestations (Line 22.6), it is recommended for **anxiety**, emotional lability, **depression**, sadness, pre-menstrual syndrome (PMS), peri-/**menopausal syndrome**, nervous exhaustion, **insomnia**, **sleepwalking** and **psychosis**.

In children, the formula can be used in cases of bed-wetting, nocturnal crying and epilepsy.

Modifications:

- Severe *qì* vacuity, + *Dang shen, Huang qì*

- Insomnia and many dreams, + *Suan zao ren, Bai zi ren*

- *Yīn* vacuity depression, insomnia, + ***Bǎi hé zhī mǔ tāng*** or ***Bǎi hé dì huáng tāng***

- Restless, easily loses temper, + ***Xiāo yáo sàn*** (see the 'Constraint pattern' section below)

- Schizophrenia, psychosis, + *Long gu, Mu li*

Like plum pit *qì*, visceral agitation is a common illness response to mental–emotional stress. The patient cannot control their crying and feelings of sadness; according to the *Inner Canon*, yawning and stretching the body balances the ascending and descending movement of *qì* and the interaction of *yīn* and *yáng*. The typical *Gān mài dà zǎo tāng* patient is overly sensitive, self-conscious and unable to focus. In the 20th century, *zàng zào* was often translated as 'hysteria' because its clinical manifestations were similar to some of the classical signs and symptoms that had been identified with the neurosis made famous by Sigmund Freud (1856–1939). (Classical hysteria signs and symptoms include hysterical blindness, paralysis, vomiting and pain; *globus hystericus*, dysphagia, dyspnoea, food dyscrasia, fainting spells, anxiety and palpitations; problems with menstrual, sexual and reproductive functions [Garvey 2001].)

躁 *Zào* means 'restlessness' and 'agitation,' and refers to the patient's feelings of distress. 脏 (藏) *Zàng* has sometimes been interpreted as the uterus, sometimes as the heart, liver or spleen visceral systems. Sometimes it is interpreted as all five *zàng* viscera, and today, source-based translators give *zàng zào* as 'visceral agitation.'

The term *zàng zào* (visceral agitation), and Zhāng Zhòngjǐng's record of its manifestations and guiding formula, all support an interpretation of the illness as a **disharmony between the *qì* of the five zàng** and their emotions. Yet, TCM textbooks usually assign visceral agitation three more specific patterns: *yīn* vacuity, heart *qì* vacuity, and heart and spleen vacuity. So, as well as or instead of *Gān mài dà zǎo tāng*, we might consider the following patterns and formula strategies, adding medicinals or modifying the prescription as needed for the *Gān mài dà zǎo tāng* patient.

The first can be a general *yīn* vacuity or a more specific **heart, lung and kidney *yīn* vacuity** pattern. Crying is the sound associated with the lung, and the lung (metal) and kidney (water) nourish each other. When the *yīn* is insufficient, empty heat disturbs the heart-*shén* which then fails to control the emotions. When the heart and kidney *yīn* in particular are depleted, the pattern is sometimes called 'heart and kidney not communicating.' The recommended formula for this illness pattern is the 'Heavenly Emperor's Tonify the Heart Pill' (天王补心丹 *Tiān wáng bǔ xīn dān*), first published in the late Ming and recommended for **exhaustion** from too much thinking.

Tiān wáng bǔ xīn dān
(Heavenly Emperor's Tonify the Heart Pill)

Sheng di huang (Radix Rehmanniae)	120g
Ren shen (Radix Ginseng)	15g
Tian men dong (Radix Asparagi)	30g
Mai men dong (Radix Ophiopogonis)	30g
Dan shen (Radix Salviae Miltiorrhizae)	15g
Fu ling (Sclerotium Poriae Cocos)	15g
Dang gui (Radix Angelicae Sinensis)	30g
Xuan shen (Radix Scrophulariae)	15g
Yuan zhi (Radix Polygalae)	15g
Wu wei zi (Fructus Schisandrae)	30g
Bai zi ren (Semen Platycladi)	30g
Suan zao ren (Semen Ziziphi Spinosae)	30g
Jie geng (Radix Platycodi)	15g
Zhu sha (Cinnabaris)^	15g

The formula anchors and calms the *shén*, nourishes heart blood, supplements the liver and kidney *yīn*, clears empty heat, harmonizes the heart-*shén* and kidney-*zhì*.

With the appropriate clinical manifestations (irritability, fatigue, palpitations, dry stool, red tongue body, thin rapid pulse), it is recommended for **insomnia** and restless sleep, **anxiety**, emotional lability—irregular crying and laughing, peri-/**menopausal syndrome**, overthinking and excess worrying, **forgetfulness**, **poor memory**, inability to concentrate, nervous exhaustion.

(^ Prohibited substance)

Modifications:

• Substitute *Long chi* or *Zhen zhu* for *Zhu sha*^

The second pattern is **heart *qì* vacuity**. The pattern and its patho-mechanisms are explained by the five-phase controlling influence: when depleted heart *qì* (fire phase) fails to control the lung (metal phase) the patient experiences sorrow and sadness, the emotion associated with the lung. Sūn Sīmiǎo's (d. 682) 'Settle the Emotions Pill' (定志丸 *Dìng zhì wán*) addresses the heart *qì* deficiency pattern.

Dìng zhì wán (Settle the Emotions Pill)

Ren shen (Radix Ginseng)	9g
Fu ling (Sclerotium Poriae Cocos)	9g
Shi chang pu (Rhizoma Acori Tatarinowii)	9g
Yuan zhi (Radix Polygalae)	9g

The formula strengthens heart *qì* and calms the *shén*, releases constraint, opens the apertures and dislodges phlegm.

Dìng zhì wán is recommended for patients who are **fearful** and easily frightened, disheartened, **forgetful**, sad and crying for no reason. It may be used for cases presenting with incessant crying and/or laughter, **insomnia** or frequent waking, **nightmares**, palpitations, **anxiety** and panic attacks, **depression**, including postpartum depression.

Modifications:

- Insomnia, + *Suan zao ren, Fŭ shen*

- Depression, + *He huan pi*

- With heart blood vacuity, + *Dang gui, Long yan rou, Suan zao ren*

- With gallbladder *qì* vacuity, + *Fŭ shen, Long gu* (and see *Ān shén dìng zhì wán* below in the Insomnia section)

The third TCM pattern is one of **depleted *qì* and blood damaging the heart and spleen** relationship. The heart blood and spleen *qì* are often depleted by worry and excess thinking, and from the late Ming period, 'Restore the Spleen Decoction' (归脾汤 *Guī pí tāng*) is the flagship formula for this dual pattern.

Guī pí tāng (Restore the Spleen Decoction)

Ren shen (Radix Ginseng)	6g
Huang qi (Radix Astragali)	12g
Bai zhu (Rhizoma Atractylodis Macrocephalae)	12g
Dang gui (Radix Angelicae Sinensis)	12g
Long yan rou (Arillus Longan)	12g
Suan zao ren (Semen Zizyphi Spinosae)	12g
Fu ling (Sclerotium Poriae Cocos)	12g
Yuan zhi (Radix Polygalae)	12g
Mu xiang (Radix Aucklandiae)^	6g
Sheng jiang (Radix Zingiberis Recens)	3g
Zhi gan cao (honey-fried Radix Glycyrrhizae)	3g
Da zao (Fructus Jujubae)	3 pieces

The formula strengthens spleen *qi* and nourishes heart blood.

With the appropriate clinical manifestations, it is recommended for **forgetfulness** and poor concentration, **anxiety** and panic attacks, palpitations, **fearfulness**, dream-disturbed sleep, **insomnia**, menstrual disorders, withdrawal **depression**.

(^ CITES Critically endangered)[152]

Modifications:

- Substitute *Sha ren* or *Qìng pi* for *Mu xiang*^

- Forgetfulness, + *Shi chang pu*

- Anxiety and depression, + *Chai hu* and *Bai shao*

Any of these three TCM patterns might contribute to a disharmony between all five *zàng*. *Yīn* vacuity can lead to disharmony due to malnourishment of the heart-*shén*, which then fails to control the emotions. Insufficiency of the heart *yīn*, *qì* or blood means that the heart-*shén* is unable to govern the five *shén* and their associated *zàng*, sensory,

---

152 CITES: the Convention on International Trade in Endangered Species of Wild Fauna and Flora, is an international treaty and agreement between governments to protect endangered plants and animals

cognitive and emotional activities. All four of these formula strategies may therefore be considered for the *zàng zào* visceral agitation patient:

- **Gān mài dà zǎo tāng** for disharmony between the five *zàng*.

- **Tiān wáng bǔ xīn tāng** for heart and kidney *yīn* deficiency.

- **Dìng zhì wán** for heart *qì* deficiency.

- **Guī pí tāng** for depleted blood and *qì* of the heart and spleen.

Careful analysis of the diagnostic data to determine the patho-mechanisms at work will identify the primary illness pattern and appropriate therapeutic reponse.

When considering the *Gān mài dà zǎo tāng* formula strategy, it is important to remember that its ingredients are not especially well known for nourishing *yīn*-fluids or supplementing the heart and spleen. Its powerful effect for disordered *shén* illnesses appears instead to be due to its gentle simplicity. The patho-mechanism is related to five-phase cycles of engendering and restraint and the balance of *qì*. The combined flavor and nature of its three ingredients overall are sweet and mild, *qì* qualities that soften, harmonize and relax the *qì* of the five *zàng*.

Running piglet qì disease

Running piglet *qì* disease (奔豚气病 *bēn tún qì bìng*) is the main illness category discussed in Chapter 8 of the *Golden Cabinet*. 'Running piglet *qì*' is the ancient name for an illness characterized by the feeling of disorderly *qì* ascending from the lower abdomen to the chest and throat, like running piglets.

> [Line 8.1] Running piglet *qì* disease refers to a surging from the lower jiāo to the throat. During attacks, the patient feels they are about to die; then the *qì* returns and the disease stops. This comes from fright.

The derangement of *qì* and the upsurging sensation are due to mental–emotional injury caused by **fright**, **fear** or **anger**. The patient feels extremely uncomfortable and often reports they feel they might die. Accompanying signs and symptoms are likely to include lower abdominal pain, especially during onset, with palpitations, vexation, rapid breathing and dizziness.

In Western psychology, this cluster of signs and symptoms is a 'panic attack.' Panic attacks are sudden periods of severe fear or fright that may last for just a few minutes or up to an hour. The patient experiences palpitations and chest pain, with shortness of breath, shaking, sweating, numbness, feelings of dread and fear of losing control. These intense episodes are related to **anxiety** and **panic** disorders.

According to Chinese medicine, sudden emotions cause the *qì* to become disorderly and, in addition, fear causes the *qì* to descend, anger causes the *qì* to rise and fright causes the *qì* to become chaotic. Sudden disorderly *qì* movement upsets the heart-*shén* and causes palpitations; disorderly descending fails to protect the exterior and to hold closed the lower openings, so cold sweat leaks out from the body surface and in severe cases there may be urinary and fecal incontinence. It is very important that treatment addresses these patho-mechanisms. If the patient does not properly recover, disorderly descending becomes a hidden pathogenic factor that can arise when for any reason their *qì* is disturbed. In severe cases, the patient can die from fright and fear.

TCM analysis emphasizes involvement of the liver, kidney and thoroughfare vessel[153] due to the patho-mechanisms of constraint, disorderly *qì* movement and counterflow. The running piglet *qì* syndrome has two main types: one is the upsurging of *yīn* cold *qì* and is related to the heart and kidney channels; the other is related to liver *qì* constraint and an ascending counterflow of channel *qì* fire. In the *Golden Cabinet*, Zhāng Zhòngjǐng first describes the indications and strategy for *Bēn tún tāng*.

[Line 8.2] For running piglet with *qì* surging up into the chest, abdominal pain, and alternating aversion to cold and heat, 'Running Piglet Decoction' (奔豚汤 *Bēn tún tāng*) governs.

Bēn tún tāng (Running Piglet Decoction)

Gan cao (Radix Glycyrrhizae)		6g
Chuan xiong (Rhizoma Chuanxiong)		6g
Dang gui (Radix Angelicai Sinensis)		6g
Ban xia (Rhizoma Pinelliae)		12g
Huang qin (Radix Scutellariae)		6g

---

153 The thoroughfare vessel (冲脉 *chōng mài*) is one of Chinese medicine's eight extraordinary vessels

Sheng ge (Radix Puerariae Cruda) (Ge gen) 15g

Bai shao (Radix Paeoniae) 6g

Sheng jiang (Rhizoma Zingiberis Recens) 12g

Gan li gen bai pi (Cortex Pruni Salicinae
Radicus) (*Sang bai pi*) 12g

The formula nourishes blood, soothes the liver, harmonizes the stomach and restores *qì* descending. It moves blood and relaxes tension to relieve pain, and helps drain the heart.

With the appropriate clinical manifestations (as described in Lines 8.1 and 8.2), *Bēn tún tāng* is recommended for **anxiety**, extreme anxiety, panic disorder, **phobias** and fearfulness, **depression**, major depression, **psychosis** and schizophrenia.

Bēn tún tāng is best suited to running piglet *qì* presenting with heat signs. It clears heat and drains the heart, nourishes blood and relaxes the liver, and it restores the descending movement of *qì*. For the *yīn*-cold type of upsurging *qì*, the main formula strategies are:

- **Guì zhī jiā guì tāng** for heart *yáng* vacuity (see the *Golden Cabinet*, Line 8.3 and the case discussion in Chapter 9)

and

- **Guì zhī jiā lóng gǔ mǔ lì tāng** for depleted *yīn* and *yáng*, and loss of essence. We discuss *Guì zhī jiā lóng gǔ mǔ lì tāng* in the next illness category, 'depletion taxation.'

Depletion taxation

Zhāng Zhòngjǐng introduced the 'depletion taxation' (虚劳 *xū láo*)[154] illness category in Chapter 6 of the *Golden Cabinet*. Depletion taxation is a serious and potentially life-threatening disorder characterized by weakness and debility. While not a psychological illness category, severe depletion illness patterns can disrupt *shén zhì* functions. Therefore, the mechanisms of disruption described by Zhāng Zhòngjǐng and some of his Chapter 6 formula strategies can be applied in some

---

154 虚劳 *Xū láo*, a disease name for severe weakness, debility and exhaustion, is also translated as 'deficiency taxation,' 'deficiency fatigue' and 'asthenia fatigue'

cases of mental–emotional illness. *Guì zhī jiā lóng gǔ mǔ lì tāng* is an example.

Line 6.3 says that depleted *yīn* essence and *yáng qì* is a common form of depletion taxation. In men, it is mainly due to excess sexual intercourse damaging and consuming the *yīn* essence, and leading to sterility.

[Line 6.8] If patients suffering from seminal loss present with uncomfortable tension in the lower abdomen and cold genitals, blurred vision, hair loss and a pulse that is extremely forceless…this means seminal loss in men or night-time dreaming of intercourse in women. 'Cinnamon Twig plus Dragon Bone and Oyster Shell Decoction' (桂枝加龙骨牡蛎汤 *Guì zhī jiā lóng gǔ mǔ lì tāng*) governs.

Guì zhī jiā lóng gǔ mǔ lì tāng (Cinnamon Twig plus Dragon Bone and Oyster Shell Decoction)

Gui zhi (Ramulus Cinnamomi)	9g
Bai shao yao (Radix Paeoniae)	9g
Sheng jiang (Rhizoma Zingibeis Recens)	9g
Gan cao (Radix Glycyrrhizae)	6g
Da zao (Fructus Jujubae)	12 pieces
Long gu (Mastodi Ossis Fossilia)	30g
Mu li (Ostreae Concha)	30g

The formula astringes the *jīng*-essence and anchors floating *yáng*, strengthens *yáng* and supplements *yīn*, restores the *qì* dynamic, and harmonizes the heart and kidneys, the (营卫) *yíng wèi*, *yīn* and *yáng*.

With appropriate clinical presentations (see Line 6.8), the formula may apply to cases of **depression** (including postpartum depression), **fearfulness**, phobias, nervousness and excitability, **anxiety** and **panic attack** disorders, lassitude, **psychosis**, mania, PMS, **insomnia**, dream-disturbed sleep, nightmares, peri-/**menopausal syndrome**, epilepsy, **forgetfulness**, weariness, nervous exhaustion, hair loss, post-traumatic stress disorder (PTSD), male infertility, erectile dysfunction.

In children: pale and emaciated with night sweating, bed-wetting, night terrors, cries easily, developmental delays, sparse thin hair, convulsions, epilepsy.

The formula improves the body condition and calms the mind. It restores and harmonizes **depleted *yīn* and *yáng*** in both women and men. It addresses a state when insufficient *yīn* affects the *yáng*: when *yáng* cannot secure the *yīn*, there is seminal emission; when *yáng* is not nourished by *yīn*, it floats and causes dreaming of sex. **Floating *yáng*** can manifest with a subjective feeling of upward movement, throbbing or palpitations in the chest and abdomen. Dizziness and hair loss are due to depleted *jīng*-blood, the *yīn* essences. The patient is nervous, overly sensitive and easily startled. They often report having insomnia with dreams and their overall pulse will be large and forceless.

In the *Golden Cabinet*, the origin of the condition is due to insufficiency of *yīn* from excess sexual activity and seminal emission during dreams. As well, or alternatively, the *yīn* has been damaged by blood loss or watery diarrhea with undigested food. In practice, severely depleted *yīn* and *yáng* can also occur due to overwork and other forms of exhaustion.

External cold damage causing severe damage to the spleen and stomach accounts for another form of depletion taxation. Zhāng Zhòngjǐng addresses this in Line 6.13. His description of the illness explains that the patient has abdominal pain that feels better with warmth, digestive problems, fatigue and aching limbs. This type of depletion taxation can result from external cold damage, overwork, chronic illness, poor diet, or poor recovery from serious illnesses, including eating disorders. In these cases, Zhāng's guiding formulas are the center-fortifying formulas.

Depletion taxation from damage to the spleen and stomach *yáng qì* is not considered a mental–emotional illness and the center-fortifying formulas are not *shén zhì bìng* formulas. Even so, Zhāng explains how the depleted earth phase (spleen and stomach) drains its mother, the fire phase (the heart), causing the patient to experience signs and symptoms of **shén–yì disharmony**: vexation and palpitations indicate that the heart-*shén* is affected. The *Golden Cabinet*'s center-fortifying formulas strengthen and warm the middle *jiāo* to produce *qì* and blood, the postnatal *qì* substances that support and harmonize depleted *yīn* essence and *yáng qì*.

[Line 6.13] In depletion taxation with abdominal urgency, palpitations, spontaneous external bleeding, pain in the abdomen, seminal loss while dreaming, aching pain in the limbs, vexing heat in the hands and feet, and dry throat and mouth, 'Minor Center-Fortifying Decoction' (小建中汤 *Xiǎo jiàn zhōng tāng*) governs.

Xiǎo jiàn zhōng tāng
(Minor Center-Fortifying Decoction)

Gui zhi (Ramulus Cinnamomi)	9g
Gan cao (Radix Glycyrrhizae)	6g
Da zao (Fructus Jujubae)	12 pieces
Bai shao (Radix Paeoniae)	18g
Sheng jiang (Rhizoma Zingiberis Recens)	9g
Yi tang (Maltosum)	30g

The formula warms and strengthens the spleen and stomach, relieves pain, supplements blood to nourish the heart, tonifies *qì* and blood and harmonizes *yīn* and *yáng*.

With appropriate clinical presentations (as in Line 6.13), the formula may apply in cases of chronic and intermittent epigastric and abdominal pain, chronic gastritis, poor appetite, **eating disorders**, palpitations, **insomnia**, irritability and restlessness, **depression** and IBS.

In children, the formula can be used in cases of poor constitution, thin build, bed-wetting, night-crying, headache, fussy eaters, hyperactivity disorders, poor appetite and constipation.

Modifications:

- For similar symptoms clusters, with spontaneous sweating, numbness or insensitivity due to severely depleted *qì* damaging the lung-*pò*, + *Huang qì* = ***Huáng qí jiàn zhōng tāng***

- For postpartum emaciation, weakness and depression, + *Dang gui* = ***Dāng guī jiàn zhōng tāng*** (see 'Postpartum Depression and Psychosis' in the 'Contemporary illness categories' section on the following pages)

The constraint syndrome

The 'constraint syndrome' (郁证 *yù zhèng*) has been linked to mental–emotional disorders since the Song, Jin and Yuan period (960–1368), and especially since the Qing (1662–1911). Today, 郁 *yù* is part of the modern Chinese word for sadness and melancholy (忧郁 *yōu yù*) and the Chinese term for clinical depression (抑郁 *yì yù*). However, our current use of *yù*-constraint for illness patterns due to internal (mental–emotional) factors is the reverse of its original meaning in the *Inner Canon*. In the *Elementary Questions*, 郁 *yù* is the term for blockages and accumulations due to external (climatic) factors.

Chinese medicine has several terms for impeded movement: for example, 'stasis' (瘀 *yū*) for static blood; 'cover' (蔽 *bì*) for obstructions that cover the sense apertures; and 'stagnation' (滞 *zhì*) for the inhibited movement of food or *qì*, such as in the liver *qì* stagnation pattern. For the *Inner Canon*'s authors, orderly *qì* movement and functions facilitated physical, mental and emotional wellbeing, and they explained how external, internal and pathogenic factors could constrain the *qì* and lead to various types of disruption. However, *yù*-constraint was not a feature of medical discourses again until the Song and Yuan dynasties when Chén Yán (1131–1189) and Zhū Dānxī (1281–1358) re-examined the idea and its role in many illness processes.

From the Song dynasty, the pathogenic potential of prolonged or immoderate mental–emotional states moved into the foreground. While Chén Yán pointed out the importance of *qì* constraint due to emotional factors, Zhū Dānxī argued that *qì* constraint could cause or accompany other forms of stagnation. His *yù*-constraint pattern included six sub-categories—the **stagnation of *qì*, dampness, fire, mucus, blood** and **food**. As a guide for their treatment, he formulated the 'Escape Restraint Pill' (越鞠丸 *Yuè jū wán*).

Yuè jū wán (Escape Restraint Pill)

Cang zhu (Rhizoma Atractylodis)	9g
Chuan xiong (Rhizoma Chuanxiong)	9g
Xiang fu (Rhizoma Cyperi)	9g
Zhi zi (Fructus Gardeniae)	9g
Shen qu (Massa Medicate Fermentata)	9g

To release constraint, the formula ingredients address the six factors that inhibit *qì* movement: they dry dampness, move blood, course the liver *qì*, clear heat and restore the middle burner's ascending and descending *qì* dynamic.

With appropriate clinical manifestations (such as stuffiness in the chest and diaphragm, rib-side discomfort or pain, distending pain in the epigastric or abdominal regions, poor appetite with belching), the formula may be appropriate for cases of **plum pit *qì***, gastric neurosis, IBS, **psychosis**, **anxiety**, **depression**.

The formula is designed to be modified so that its ability to transform and resolve all forms of constraint can target individual patient presentations and patho-mechanisms.

Modifications:

- Mental–emotional (psychological) disorders with

    - Static blood, + *Hong hua*

    - Phlegm dampness, + *Zhi ban xia* or *Fǔ ling*

    - Fire, + *Qing dai*

    - *Qì* stagnation, + *Qing pi* or increase the doseage of *Xiang fǔ*

    - Liver *qì* constraint, + *Chai hu* and *Bai shao*

- Plum pit *qì* (*globus hystericus*), + *Yu jin* or *Hou pò* or *Ji nei jīng*, or *Er chen tāng*

Chén Yán and Zhū Dānxī re-established the importance and dynamics of mental–emotional factors for internal disorders. Then in the Ming, Zhào Xiànkě[155] (1572–1643) explained how the processes of stagnation and constraint led to pathogenic fire. Zhào's representation of constraint as an obstruction of physiological fire, however, took him on a different course from Chén Yán and Zhū Dānxī and their strategies for draining repletion fire illness states.

In cases of constraint with pathogenic fire, Zhào did not prescribe harsh medicinals to clear fire and disperse the stagnation. Instead, he unblocked the constraint more gently by supporting and **harmonizing the *qì* and blood**. His approach is best represented by his use of the

---

155 赵献可 Zhào Xiànkě

Song dynasty formula 'Free Wanderer Powder' (逍遥散 *Xiāo yáo sàn*) (Scheid 2013).

Xiāo yáo sàn (Free Wanderer Powder)

Chai hu (Radix Bupleuri)	9g
Chao dang gui (dry-fried Radix Angelicae Sinensis)	9g
Bai shao (Radix Paeoniae Alba)	9g
Bai zhu (Rhizoma Atractylodis Macrocephalae)	9g
Fu ling (Sclerotium Poriae Cocos)	9g
Zhi gan cao (prepared Radix Glycyrrhizae)	4.5g
Wei jiang (baked Rhizoma Zingiberis Recens)	6g
Bo he (Menthae Haplocalycis)	3g

The formula harmonizes the liver and spleen to release *qì* constraint. It soothes the liver, strengthens the spleen, regulates *qì* and supplements blood.

With the appropriate clinical manifestations (poor or irregular appetite, rib-side, chest or abdominal fullness and distending pain, which are worse with mental, emotional stress, and fine wiry pulse), *Xiāo yáo sàn* may be applied in cases of **insomnia**, **anxiety**, poor appetite, PMS, **menstrual disorders**, fatigue, peri-/**menopausal syndrome**, irritability, despondency, **depression**, pent-up frustration.

Modifications:

- When stagnation and constraint transform into pathogenic fire, + *Zhi zi* and *Mu dan pi* = ***Jiā wèi xiāo yáo sàn***

Anger and frustration are the liver *zāng*'s associated emotions and temperament. The liver and its disposition are both *yáng* in nature and because of this, liver *qì* constraint easily transforms into pathogenic fire. Fire constraint patterns especially affect the liver and gallbladder, heart and pericardium. Fire constraint can cause, exacerbate or accompany other illness patterns such as blood stasis, phlegm dampness, damp heat or phlegm heat, and various depletion patterns, in which case more complex treatment strategies may be needed.

Xiāo yáo sàn is a famous modification of two Zhāng Zhòngjǐng formulas: 'Frigid Extremities Powder' (四逆散 *Sì nì sàn*, from the

Treatise on Cold Damage), and 'Danggui and Peony Powder' (当归芍药散 *Dāng guī sháo yào sàn*) from the *Golden Cabinet*. *Sì nì sàn* treats **liver *qì* 'stagnation'** (滞 *zhì*), a repletion pattern where *qì* stagnation traps the *yáng qì* in the interior and prevents it reaching the extremities. Because *Sì nì sàn* restores liver free coursing and orderly reaching, it helps to relieve mental–emotional stress and the bodily symptoms caused by stress.

Sì nì sàn (Frigid Extremities Powder)

Chai hu (Radix Bupleuri)	12g
Bai shao yao (Radix Paeoniae)	24g
Zhi shi (Fructus Aurantii Immaturus)	12g
Zhi gan cao (prepared Radix Glycyrrhizae)	9g

The formula harmonizes the liver and spleen, relieves stagnation, spreads the liver *qì* and eliminates heat. These actions relieve mental–emotional depression.

With the appropriate clinical manifestations (cold hands and feet, fullness and distending pain in the rib-sides, chest, abdomen or stomach, wiry pulse, symptoms that worsen with stress), *Sì nì sàn* may be applied in cases of hepatitis, **depression**, PMS, **menstrual disorders**, irritability and anger, **insomnia**, peri-/**menopausal syndrome**, restlessness, **anxiety**, IBS, gastritis.

Sì nì sàn can be prescribed as is but is usually modified, combined with other formulas, or it appears as a basis for formulas such as ***Xiāo yáo sàn*** (see above), ***Chái hú shū gān sàn*** (see the section on 'Depression' following), and ***Xué fǔ zhú yu tāng*** (discussed in 'Insomnia').

Modifications:

- Chronic insomnia, + *Dang gui, Chuan xiong, Tao ren, Hong hua*

- Insomnia and excess dreams, + *Suan zao ren, Yuan zhi*

- Epigastric pain, + *Zhi shi, Zhi ke, Gan cao*

- Chest pain, + ***Bàn xià hòu pǔ tāng***

- Painful periods, + *Dang gui, Wu yao, Yan hu suo*

- Impotence and cold pain in the lower abdomen, + *Ba ji tian, Gou qi zi, Yin zhi ren*

- ***Xiāo yáo sàn*** is more appropriate for cases with signs of depletion (weakened *qi* functions, fatigue, blood vacuity)

- ***Dāng guī sháo yáo sàn*** also treats liver constraint with spleen vacuity but is more often used for gynecological disorders (it benefits the spleen and kidney and relieves pain, see 'Gynecological pain')

Orderly liver *qi* functions ensure the harmonious movement of *qi* and blood. Restoring liver free coursing in turn relaxes mental and emotional activities and responses so that the patient feels clear and positive. In the liver *qi* constraint (郁 *yù*) pattern, liver 'dredging and discharge' (疏泄 *shū xiè*) are weakened and depressed: the person is taciturn, gloomy and uncommunicative, they sigh a lot and are susceptible to doubt, confusion and pent-up frustration. In the liver *qi* stagnation (滞 *zhì*) pattern, the liver *qi* is replete and its movement impeded: the person feels physically and mentally restless, they are hot-tempered and rash and have trouble sleeping.

From the Qing (1644–1911), the *yù zhèng*-constraint pattern became not only a mechanism of disorder but an illness category, a mental–emotional disorder. From that time, it tends to be specific to the liver and due to internal injury. Furthermore, treatment required that the patient develop insight regarding their perceptions, responses and behaviors. It was Yè Tiānshì[156] (1666–1745) who proposed that healing *yù zhèng* depends on the patient's ability to transform their emotions and personality (Zhang 2007).

Yù-constraint is a major factor instigating or complicating all kinds of pathogenic changes. It may be identified in patients who are dealing with clinically diverse experiences and symptoms such as anger problems, agitation, anxiety, infertility, cystitis or irritable bowel syndrome (IBS). To treat disorders with *yù*-constraint patterns, today's Chinese medicine physicians in China include strategies to rectify liver *shū xiè* functions and often combine treatment with 'persuasion or disentanglement' (疏理 *shū lǐ*) of the patient's personal and emotional blockages (Zhang 2007).

---

156 叶天士 Yè Tiānshì

Yù zhèng clinical manifestations are varied and diverse. The patient's lived experience tends to be one of mental, emotional and physical tension, and symptoms are relieved or worsened according to their mental–emotional state. Because the liver channel runs through the sexual and reproductive organs, the digestive organs, chest, rib-sides and throat, liver *qì* constraint tends to affect these areas in particular. Common presenting problems include abdominal, chest and/or rib-side distention and pain, the sensation of plum-stone throat ('plum pit *qì*,' or *globus hystericus*), tension headaches, anger, despondency, erectile dysfunction, inability to eat, menstrual disorders and blurred vision (Garvey and Qu 2001; Yan and Li 2007).

A continued pattern of liver *qì* stagnation and constraint can transform into pathogenic fire, and pathogenic fire in turn can consume the *yīn*-blood and fluids and damage the *qì*. The liver-*hún* becomes agitated and cannot settle. When pathogenic fire accumulates in the upper *jiāo* the heart-*shén* and lung-*pò* relationships are also disrupted. The resulting manifestations are likely to include sleep disturbances, inappropriate verbal or emotional responses or laughter, absent-mindedness, forgetfulness, poor judgment and poor problem solving. These kinds of signs and symptoms were first identified in the *Golden Cabinet*, especially in relation to the **plum pit *qì*** (*Bàn xià hòu pǔ tāng*) and **visceral agitation** (*Gān mài dà zǎo tāng*) illness categories.

Regulating the liver system has become an important strategy for the treatment of depression in recent times, for all the reasons just mentioned. The liver governs free coursing, and of all the *zàng*, the liver and heart are the most immediately affected by emotional strain. The liver's upward and spreading nature resents being constrained, its channel runs through the chest, abdomen, genital and reproductive organs, and the liver-*hún* is associated with the realm of the unconscious, our dreams and visionary states.

Contemporary illness categories

Depression

In Western Chinese medicine clinics today, the 'liver constraint' (肝郁 *gān yù*) pattern is easily conflated with clinical depression. For one thing, the term 郁 *yù* is often translated as 'depression,' although its meaning is that *qì* activities are lessened and constrained. Furthermore, the term 郁 *yù*-constraint/depression describes the depressive mood that is associated with mental–emotional strain; and finally, the *yù zhèng*-constraint pattern is very common in patients presenting with depression. However, many cases of clinical depression will present with illness patterns other than liver *qì* constraint. We will come to these shortly, but first a recap of *yù zhèng*, the constraint pattern, and relevant Chinese medicine strategies for clinical depression.

In the last illness category, we discussed how *yù zhèng* caused stagnation on all levels, physical, mental and emotional. We saw how liver *qì* constraint produces a wide array of signs, symptoms and disorders, including emotional constraint or depression, and how it is linked with other forms of stagnation such as phlegm dampness and static blood, producing accumulations and lumps. One example of these patho-mechanisms is the sensation of a lump in the throat as in the section above on 'plum-pit *qì*.'

There we noted the *Golden Cabinet*'s guiding formula, **Bàn xià hòu pǔ tāng** (Pinellia and Magnolia Bark Decoction), and its suitability for patients with clinical depression. *Bàn xià hòu pǔ tāng* relieves constraint, disperses accumulations, dissolves phlegm and restores stomach *qì* downbearing. From the key symptom, plum pit *qì*, we can extrapolate to include other throat conditions, for instance persistent dryness, itching or pain in the throat. Difficulty swallowing may accompany digestive complaints such as poor appetite, nausea or a stuffy feeling in the chest and epigastric region in cases of chronic gastritis or gastro-intestinal neuroses.

The *yù zhèng*-constraint pattern can arise and develop to include a number of stagnation, depletion and repletion states affecting the *zàng shén* and their *qì* influences, and Chinese medicine has developed successful treatment strategies for various forms of liver stagnation and constraint. With appropriate presentations, these may be considered for the management of depression. Careful diagnostic differentiation is needed to identify priorities for treatment and to select appropriate formulas and modifications. As well as the *Bàn xià hòu pǔ tāng* form of constraint, we have already covered most of the other important constraint pattern formulas:

- **Yuè jū wán** (Escape Restraint Pill) is considered a guide for strategies to resolve the six constraints (*qì*, blood, phlegm, fire, dampness and food), which can easily combine and form major or contributing roles in constraint illness patterns. The formula can be modified and adapted for cases of depression, depending on individual presentations that might include anger and restlessness, chest oppression, rib-side discomfort, epigastric or abdominal distending pain, acid belching, poor appetite, irregular bowel movements and/or nausea.

- *Sì nì sàn* (Frigid Extremities Powder) is the guiding formula strategy for replete forms of liver *qì* stagnation and where cold hands and feet are a feature of the presentation. Typical accompanying signs and symptoms include distention or pain in the stomach, lower abdomen or rib-sides, alternating constipation and loose stools. Signs and symptoms will feel worse with nervousness or stress.

Though rarely used on its own, *Sì nì sàn* is often modified or incorporated into other formulas, such as:

- *Xiāo yáo sàn* (Free Wanderer Powder) *Sì nì sàn* and *Xiāo yáo sàn* both harmonize the liver and spleen. *Xiāo yáo sàn* soothes the liver to relieve constraint, strengthens the spleen and nourishes the blood. It is frequently used for mild mental–emotional disorders including depression with fatigue and tension, poor appetite, rib-side discomfort, menstrual pain and pre-menstrual syndrome (PMS).

- *Jiā wèi xiāo yáo sàn* is substituted for *Xiāo yáo sàn* in cases where constraint has transformed into pathogenic heat.

- 'Bupleurum Powder to Dredge the Liver' (柴胡疏肝汤 *Chái hú shū gān tāng*), a variation of *Sì nì sàn*'s strategy addressing **repletion *qì* constraint** patterns.

Chái hú shū gān tāng (Bupleurum Powder to Dredge the Liver)

Cu chao chen pi (vinegar-fried Pericarpium Citri Reticulatae)	6g
Chai hu (Radix Bupleuri)	6g
Chuan xiong (Rhizoma Chuanxiong)	4.5g
Bai shao yao (Radix Paeoniae)	4.5g

> *Chao zhi ke* (dry-fried Fructus Aurantii)   4.5g
>
> *Zhi gan cao* (prepared Radix Glycyrrhizae)   1.5g
>
> *Xiang fu* (Rhizoma Cyperi)   4.5g
>
> The formula soothes and spreads the liver *qì*, harmonizes the blood, relieves pain, and is recommended for emotional stress and frustrated emotions that easily give rise to anger.
>
> With the appropriate clinical manifestations (wiry pulse, stuffy feeling in the rib-sides and chest, abdominal distention, belching, sighing, symptoms worsen with stress, pain improves with exercise), *Chái hú shū gān tāng* may be applied in cases of hepatitis, **depression**, PMS, **menstrual disorders**, irritability and anger, **insomnia**, **psychosis**, IBS, chronic gastritis.

While the liver *qì* constraint pattern is a common feature in cases of depression, TCM analysis supports the diagnosis of liver *qì* constraint as a main or associated pattern for many psychological disorders, not only depression. Moreover, many patients with clinical depression do not present with liver *qì* constraint or with any liver illness pattern. Chinese medicine discourses explaining 'cold' manifestation clusters due to depleted *yáng qì* reveal another important strategy for this illness category.

During the Ming (1368–1662) and Qing (1662–1911) dynasties, scholar-physicians considered lifegate fire the force that animated the body. Its true and original *yáng* was responsible for initiating life *qì* movements and transformations. Contrary to Zhū Dānxī's representation of the nature of physiological fire as tending to excess and repletion, Ming scholar-physicians found that the kidney *yáng* and lifegate fire were just as likely to become weakened and depleted.

To strengthen depleted physiological fire and support its movement through the body, Zhāng Jièbīn[157] (1563–1640) developed the 'Right Restoring (Lifegate) Pill' (右归丸 *Yòu guī wán*).

---

157 张介宾 Zhāng Jièbīn

Yòu guī wán (Right Restoring Pill)

Zhi fu zi (prepared Radix Aconiti Lateralis)	18g
Rou gui (Cortex Cinnamomi)	12g
Lu jiao jiao (Cervi Cornus Colla)^	12g
Shu di huang (prepared Radix Rehmanniae)	24g
Shan zhu yu (Fructus Corni)	9g
Chao shan yao (dry fried Rhizoma Dioscoreae)	12g
Chao gou qì zi (dry fried Fructus Lycii Chinensis)	12g
Tu si zi (Semen Cuscutae)	12g
Du zhong (Cortex Eucommiae)	12g
Dang gui (Radix Angelicae Sinensis)	9g

The formula's principal ingredients strengthen and warm kidney *yáng*, the original *yáng* and lifegate fire.

With the appropriate clinical manifestations (indicating depleted kidney *yáng qì* with cold signs and symptoms), the formula is recommended for **depression**, somnolence, senile **dementia**, senile itching, **forgetfulness**, **menopausal syndrome**, palpitations.

(^ CITES critically endangered)

Depleted kidney *yáng*, the lifegate fire, affects all the visceral systems and their *qì* influences: the person feels weak and cold; the spleen and stomach cannot digest food; the bladder and kidney *qì* are weakened and the water passages become obstructed. These conditions produce urinary and gastro-intestinal disorders, fluid retention and diminished sexual drive. Mental–emotional activities and responses are likely to be affected—the person feels disoriented, despondent, apathetic; their reactions to external stimulus are slow and dispirited; their ability to focus, analyze, plan and decide is diminished.

In the *Golden Cabinet*, Zhāng Zhòngjǐng's discussion of depletion taxation (虚劳 *xū láo*) disorders—the severe depletions of *yīn* and *yáng*, *qì* and blood, *zàng* and *fǔ*—had already documented a response to **depleted kidney *yáng* and lifegate fire**. After the center-fortifying decoctions for spleen and stomach *yáng qì* deficiency in Lines 6.12–6.14, Line 6.15 records the indications and guiding formula for depleted kidney *yáng*, the 'Eight-ingredient Kidney *Qì* Pill' (八味肾气丸 *Bā wèi shèn qì wán*).

[Line 6.15] In depletion taxation with lumbar pain, hypertonicity in the lower abdomen and inhibited urination, 'Eight-ingredient Kidney *Qì* Pill' (八味肾气丸 *Bā wèi shèn qì wán*) governs.

Bā wèi shèn qì wán (Eight-ingredient Kidney *Qì* Pill or '*Jīn guì shèn qì wán*,' and 'Rehmania Eight')

Gan di huang (Radix Rehmanniae)	30g
Shan yao (Rhizoma Dioscoreae)	15g
Shan zhu yu (Fructus Corni)	20g
Ze xie (Rhizoma Alismatis)	15g
Fu ling (Sclerotium Poriae Cocos)	15g
Mu dan pi (Cortex Moutan)	15g
Gui zhi (Ramulus Cinnamomi)	15g
Fu zi (prepared Radix Aconiti Lateralis)	15g

The formula warms and strengthens kidney *yáng*.

With the appropriate clinical manifestations (Line 6.15), it is recommended for **depression**, somnolence, peri-/**menopausal syndrome**, **forgetfulness**, senile **dementia**, senile itching, hysterical paralysis, scanty menses and PMS.

The *Golden Cabinet*'s *Bā wèi shèn qì wán*, and Zhāng Jièbīn's *Yòu guī wán*, are both built around a group of medicinals that nourish the *yīn*, blood, essence and marrow, with the addition of *yáng*-strengthening substances. This is in line with the principle of strengthening the *yáng* (lifegate fire) within the *yīn* (kidney water).

The kidney *zàng* governs the lower back, and therefore lower back discomfort or pain is a common sign for kidney illness patterns. Lumbar pain due to insufficiency of kidney *yáng* will have a feeling of weakness that worsens with exertion and feels better with warmth. Patients with depression often have disturbed sleep. In many cases, this is lack of sleep, but depressive disorder patients frequently present with over-sleeping. *Yáng qì* vacuity tends to cause dullness, drowsiness, somnolence and over-sleeping. In these cases, *Bā wèi shèn qì wán* and *Yòu guī wán* will be more appropriate.

- Patients with insufficient and interrupted sleep are more likely to present with *yīn* deficiency illness patterns. The lily bulb formulas, ***Bǎi hé zhī mǔ tāng*** (Lily and Anemarrhena Decoction) and ***Bǎi hé dì huáng tāng*** (Lily and Rehmannia Decoction), may be considered in *yīn* deficiency cases with appropriate clinical manifestations. The lily bulb formulas nourish the heart and lung *yīn*, clear vacuity heat, and calm and harmonize the heart-*shén* and lung-*pò*, actions that restore restful sleep. As well as clinical depression, including manic depression, *bǎi hé bìng* patients will probably present with an unusually wide variety of subjective symptoms including emotional lability, erratic behavior and disorientation.

- The key manifestation for ***Gān mài dà zǎo tāng*** (the Liquorice, Wheat and Jujube Decoction for 'visceral agitation') is the tendency to sadness and crying, with frequent yawning and stretching, and so this formula is also suitable for some patients with depressive disorders. *Gān mài dà zǎo tāng* soothes, nourishes and harmonizes all the *zàng qì*, it gently quietens the heart-*shén* and relaxes tension.

Gynecological pain

The *Golden Cabinet*, Chapters 20, 21 and 22 are the beginning and foundation of TCM gynecology. They contain 40 formulas for menstrual, pregnancy, delivery and miscellaneous disorders. Chapter 22 ('Women's Miscellaneous Diseases') repeats one of the Chapter 20 ('Women's Pregnancy') formulas, one that frequently appears in contemporary discussions of psychological illnesses associated with menstruation and pregnancy.

[Line 20.5] For women's abdominal tension and pain during pregnancy, 'Chinese Angelica and Peony Powder' (当归芍药散 *Dāng guī sháo yào sàn*) governs.

[Line 22.17] For all abdominal pain in women, *Dāng guī sháo yào sàn* governs.

Dāng guī sháo yào sàn
(Chinese Angelica and Peony Powder)

Dang gui (Radix Angelicae Sinensis)	12g
Bai shao yao (Radix Paeoniae)	48g
Fu ling (Sclerotium Poriae Cocos)	12g
Bai zhu (Rhizoma Atractylodis Macrocephalae)	12g
Ze xie (Rhizoma Alismatis)	24g
Chuan xiong (Rhizoma Chuanxiong)	24g

Dāng guī sháo yào sàn is used for abdominal pain in women. It treats liver constraint with spleen vacuity, benefits the spleen and kidney, and the large dose of *Bai shao yao* relaxes tension and relieves pain.

The formula may be used in cases with appropriate clinical manifestations, namely, abdominal tension and pain, persistent cramping pain with oedema of lower legs and feet, including during pregnancy. It is recommended for menstrual disorders (scanty, delayed or painful periods), PMS, peri-/**menopausal syndrome**, senile **dementia**, postpartum **depression**, palpitations, lassitude.

Tension and continuous dull pain in the abdomen are the identifying symptoms for this kind of **liver and spleen disharmony** (a form of **vacuity *qì* constraint**). The formula nourishes liver blood to relieve constraint, relaxes tension, de-obstructs *qì* and blood, strengthens the spleen and resolves dampness.

During pregnancy, blood gathers to nourish the foetus, and overall blood becomes relatively depleted. Not only in pregnancy but whenever liver blood is insufficient, the liver's orderly 'dredging and discharge' (疏泄 *shū xiè*) functions are impaired. At this point, emotional stress can cause the liver *qì* to invade the spleen, creating abdominal pain associated with menstruation or menopause, or during pregnancy. By harmonizing the liver and spleen, the formula addresses the patho-mechanisms frequently caused by internal damage due to mental–emotional stress.

Postpartum depression and psychosis
Postpartum psychological diseases begin soon after childbirth and can last from six months to a year. The symptoms of postpartum

depression include extreme sadness with crying, anxiety, irritability and low energy. The woman may experience changes in sleeping or eating patterns. Postpartum psychosis is an uncommon but very serious condition. The patient is likely to experience severe depression and confusion, with paranoia, hallucinations and delusions. Symptoms vary, can change quickly and are at their most severe from onset in the first week or two after childbirth and then up to about three months.

Zhāng Zhòngjǐng's *Golden Cabinet* recommends 'Major Order the *Qì* Decoction' (大承气汤 *Dà chéng qì tāng*) for postpartum lochia, with symptoms of delirium and agitation.

[Line 21.7] If on the seventh or eighth day after giving birth a woman has no *tàiyáng* signs, but hardness and pain in the lower abdomen, this means incomplete elimination of lochia. If accompanied by constipation, vexation, agitation and feverishness, the pulse slightly forceful, a worsening of feverishness and agitation in the late afternoon with inability to eat, delirious speech, and then relief in the evening, 'Major Order the *Qì* Decoction' (大承气汤 *Dà chéng qì tāng*) governs.

Dà chéng qì tāng (Major Order the *Qì* Decoction)

Da huang (Radix et Rhizoma Rhei) (added near the end) 12g

Mang xiao (Sulfaf Natrii) (dissolve in strained decoction) 12g

Zhi zhi shi (prepared Fructus Aurantii Immaturus)   15g

Zhi hou po (prepared Cortex Magnoliae Officinalis)   24g

This is a strong formula to drain **internal repletion heat**, which agitates the heart-*shén* causing delirium and mania.

With appropriate presenting manifestations (abdominal pain and fullness, agitation, rapid and forceful pulse), the formula may be used for cases of postpartum constipation, postpartum retention of lochia with delirious speech, **mania, psychosis**, agitation, **insomnia**, vivid dreams.

Modifications:

- For a similar illness presentation with static blood, a variation on the *Chéng qì tāng* strategy may be used, such as '**Peach Pit Order the *Qì* Decoction**' (桃核承气汤 *Táo hé chéng qì tāng*).

> ### *Táo hé chéng qì tāng* (Peach Pit Order the *Qì* Decoction)
>
> | | |
> |---|---|
> | *Tao ren* (Seman Persicae) | 15g |
> | *Da huang* (Radix et Rhizoma Rhei) (added near the end) | 12g |
> | *Gui zhi* (Ramulus Cinnamomi) | 9g |
> | *Mang xiao* (Sulfaf Natrii) (dissolve in strained decoction) | 9g |
> | *Zhi gan cao* (prepared Radix Glycyrrhizae) | 6g |
>
> This is a strong formula to break up static blood and drain internal heat accumulations.
>
> With appropriate presenting manifestations (acute severe lower abdominal pain, feverishness worse in afternoon or at night, red dry tongue, deep and forceful or choppy pulse), the formula may be used for cases of difficult birth or stillbirth, postpartum constipation, postpartum retention of lochia with delirious speech, **mania**, **psychosis**, agitation, emotional lability, peri-/**menopausal syndrome**, vivid dreams, **insomnia**, palpitations, irritability, bi-polar disorder.

Chapter 21 of the *Golden Cabinet* advises the use of 'Minor Bupleurum Decoction' (小柴胡汤 *Xiǎo chái hú tāng*) in cases of postpartum vexing heat from exposure to wind, and in cases of **postpartum constraint** with dizziness and blurred vision due to blood vacuity. As well as blood loss after giving birth, female patients may have copious sweating during and after delivery. This weakens their *yíng–wèi* and leaves them vulnerable to an attack by external wind. *Xiǎo chái hú tāng*'s harmonizing action addresses these conditions.

> ### *Xiǎo chái hú tāng* (Minor Bupleurum Decoction)
>
> | | |
> |---|---|
> | *Chai hu* (Radix Bupleuri) | 24g |
> | *Huang qìn* (Radix Scutellariae) | 15g |
> | *Zhi ban xia* (prepared Rhizoma Pinelliae) | 24g |
> | *Sheng jiang* (Rhizoma Zingiberis Recens) | 9g |
> | *Ren shen* (Radix Ginseng) | 19g |
> | *Zhi gan cao* (honey-fried Radix Glycyrrhizae) | 9g |
> | *Da zao* (Fructus Jujube) | 9g |
>
> The formula addresses clinical presentations where at regular intervals chills alternate with periods of feverishness with vexation.

> With the appropriate clinical manifestations (dry mouth and throat, bitter taste, blurred vision, restlessness, poor appetite, distending fullness in the chest and rib-sides, wiry pulse), the formula may be used for **depression, psychosis, postpartum fever**, PMS, peri-/ **menopausal syndrome**, irritability, **insomnia**, IBS.

We have already seen how stagnation and disharmony patterns were sometimes associated with the potentially life-threatening conditions of depletion taxation (虚劳 *xū láo*). The *Golden Cabinet* Chapter 6 ('Blood Impediment and Depletion Wasting') explains how the weakened earth phase (spleen and stomach) drains the fire phase (heart) and damages the heart-*shén*, leading to agitation and palpitations.

In Chinese medicine, the blood achieves many essential physiological tasks, including that of nourishing and holding the *shén*. The heart-*shén* and liver-*hún* in particular rely on the *yīn*-blood for their mental–emotional activities and responses. Treatments for women experiencing postpartum psychological disorders, such as postpartum depression, will vary to address the presenting signs and symptoms and relevant pathomechanisms. In cases where there is fatigue, palpitations, agitation, depression, insomnia and abdominal pain relieved by warmth, another of the center-fortifying formula family is indicated: 'Dang Gui Center-Fortifying Decoction' (当归建中汤 *Dāng guī jiàn zhōng tāng*).

Dāng guī jiàn zhōng tāng (Dang Gui Center-Fortifying Decoction)

Dang gui (Radix Angelica Sinensis)	9g
Gui zhi (Ramulus Cinnamomi)	9g
Gan cao (Radix Glycyrrhizae)	6g
Da zao (Fructus Jujube)	5 pieces
Bai shao (Radix Paeoniae Alba)	15g
Sheng jiang (Rhizoma Zingiberis Recens)	6g
Yi tang (Maltose)	30g

The formula warms and strengthens the middle *jiāo*, and supplements the blood to relieve pain.

With appropriate clinical manifestations, it can be used for postpartum weakness and emaciation, lassitude, persistent abdominal pain, palpitations, **insomnia**, poor appetite, **depression** and **psychosis**, including postpartum depression and psychosis.

Dāng guī jiàn zhōng tāng is a modification of Zhāng Zhòngjǐng's center-fortifying strategy, and was first recorded by Sūn Sīmiǎo[158] for cases of **postpartum emaciation and weakness**. The addition of *Dāng guī* subtly shifts the *Xiǎo jiàn zhōng tāng* formula's emphasis towards nourishing and harmonizing the blood—an important therapeutic strategy for women after childbirth (Wilms 2002). Sūn's simple and elegant modification ensures that the treatment priority, nourishing blood, is supported by warming and strengthening the middle *qì*, and harmonizing *yīn* and *yáng*.

Sūn Sīmiǎo's encyclopaedic collection, the *Priceless and Essential Formulas for Emergencies*[159] (652), contains Chinese medicine's first detailed analysis of women's menstrual, gynecological and obstetric disorders. He understood the physical and psychological implications of *qì* and blood depletions, and recorded the potential dangers from the loss of blood after childbirth. Sūn warned of, the '**instability of the *hún* and *pò*,**' and noted important identifying manifestations: emaciation, palpitations, mental confusion, dimmed eyesight, numbness, seizures, **hallucinations** and **insanity**. Later, Fù Qīngzhǔ[160] expressed similar concerns regarding postpartum blood loss, and the 'absence of governance in the heart [*shén*] and *hún* as if walking amidst the clouds in the sky' (Fǔ 1996 [originally, 1826]).

In 1973, the distinguished clinician, reformer and modernizer of Chinese medicine, Yuè Měizhōng,[161] applied Zhāng Zhòngjǐng's analysis to his treatment of a woman with severe blood loss after giving birth (Yuè 2007). Her continuous bleeding was eventually stopped through the use of an ice bag for six hours, but by then she was in a state of extreme blood vacuity, losing consciousness and suffering with generalized palsy that was not responding to treatment. Loss of consciousness and paralysis with weakness and numbness, clearly indicate *shén* disorder, and Dr. Yuè identified her condition as a typical case of 'blood impediment.' Accordingly, he prescribed the first of the formulas presented in the *Golden Cabinet* Chapter 6, 'Blood Impediment and Depletion Taxation.'

[Line 6.2] In blood impediment, when *yīn* and *yáng* are both weak, when the pulse is faint, small and tight, and when the external signs

---

158 孙思邈 Sūn Sīmiǎo (581–682)
159 《千金要方》 *Qiān jīn yào fang*
160 傅青主 Fù Qīngzhǔ (1607–1684)
161 岳美中 Yuè Měizhōng (1900–1982)

are generalized numbness and an appearance as in wind impediment, 'Astragalus and Cinnamon Twig Five Substances Decoction' (黄芪桂枝五物汤 *Huáng qí guì zhī wǔ wù tāng*) governs.

Huáng qí guì zhī wǔ wù tāng
(Astragalus and Cinnamon Twig Five Substance Decoction)

Huang qì (Radix Astragali)	30g
Bai shao yao (Radix Paeoniae)	30g
Gui zhi (Ramulus Cinnamomi)	12g
Sheng jiang (Rhizoma Zingiberis Recens)	18g
Da zao (Fructus Jujubae)	12 pieces

The formula strenthens *qì*, supplements blood, warms the channels and the middle *jiāo*, dispels cold and unblocks painful obstruction. It harmonizes *yīn* and *yáng* by strengthening and regulating the spleen and stomach, by nourishing the blood while warming and strengthening the body, and by harmonizing the nutritive and defense (*yíng–wèi*) *qì*.

With appropriate clinical manifestations (Line 6.2), the formula is recommended for postpartum emaciation and debility, **insomnia**, palpitations, difficulty breathing, irritability, **depression**, facial tics, diabetic neuropathy, aphasia, peripheral neuritis, paresthesia, paralysis, numbness.

In their prescriptions, Sūn Sīmiǎo, Fù Qīngzhǔ and Yuè Měizhōng assimilate and deploy theoretical developments from the early classics and later periods. In the context of mental–emotional disorders, Chinese medicine methods can settle the heart-*shén* and harmonize the five *zàng shén*. By regulating *yīn* and *yáng*, and supplementing *qì* and blood, the patient's awareness, reception and management of sensory information are restored. In so doing, their cognitive activities, emotional responses and inner life become clearer and more balanced.

Menopausal syndrome

Menopause is a normal life stage when, at around the age of 50, women experience a decrease in hormone production that causes the cessation of the menses. The menopausal syndrome is a cluster of signs and symptoms that may occur during the time when menstruation changes and then stops. Common physical symptoms include hot flushes, fatigue, sore joints and weight gain. Common psychological symptoms include mood changes, difficulty sleeping, anxiety, depression, poor concentration and poor memory. Similar signs and symptoms occurring before the cessation of the menses are termed 'peri-menopausal.'

A number of the formulas already presented may be considered for patients with mental–emotional disorders associated with peri-menopausal and menopausal changes:

- *Bǎi hé zhī mǔ tāng* (Lily Combination) boosts *qì*, nourishes the *yīn* and clears *yīn* vacuity heat to settle and harmonize the heart-*shén* and lung-*pò*. With appropriate clinical presentations (see the *Golden Cabinet*, Line 3.1), *Bǎi hé zhī mǔ tāng* may apply to patients with **menopausal syndrome**, irritability and mental disorientation, clinical **depression** and **anxiety** disorders, obsessiveness, **insomnia**, **sleepwalking**, erratic behavior and mood swings.

- *Guì zhī jiā lóng gǔ mǔ lì tāng* (Cinnamon Twig Decoction plus Dragon Bone and Oyster Shell) astringes the *jīng*-essence and anchors floating *yáng*, strengthens *yáng* and supplements *yīn*, harmonizes heart and kidneys and the *yíng–wèi*. With appropriate clinical presentations (see the *Golden Cabinet*, Line 6.8), the formula may apply to patients who are **fearful**, overly sensitive and easily startled, and to cases of peri-menopausal and **menopausal syndrome**, **depression**, **anxiety** and panic attack disorders, lassitude, **psychosis**, mania, **insomnia**, nightmares, palpitations, **forgetfulness** and nervous exhaustion.

- *Bàn xià hòu pǔ tāng* (Pinellia and Magnolia Bark Decoction) transforms phlegm, dissipates clumps, benefits the stomach and spleen, releases constraint and restores the *qì* dynamic. With the appropriate clinical manifestations (as in the *Golden Cabinet* Line 22.5), the formula is recommended for peri-menopausal and **menopausal syndrome**, **plum pit *qì***, **anxiety**, excess worrying, **depression, insomnia, psychosis**, IBS, epilepsy and vomiting.

- *Gān mài dà zǎo tāng* (Liquorice, Wheat, and Jujube Decoction) harmonizes the emotions and the *qì* of the five *zàng*; it settles and harmonizes the five *shén*, regulates the middle *qì* and relaxes tension. With the appropriate clinical manifestations (see the *Golden Cabinet* Line 22.6), it is recommended for peri-menopausal and **menopausal syndrome**, nervous exhaustion, **anxiety, depression, insomnia, sleepwalking, psychosis**, emotional lability, sadness and poor concentration. For menopausal syndrome patients, *Gān mài dà zǎo tāng* may be suitable on its own, or in combination with, for example, the 'Minor Bupleurum Decoction' (小柴胡汤 *Xiǎo chái hú tāng*).

- *Xiǎo chái hú tāng* (Minor Bupleurum Decoction) releases constraint where signs and symptoms have a periodic or inter-mittent presentation. Appropriate clinical symptoms include nausea and poor appetite, rib-side distention or pain, bitter or metallic taste in the mouth, dry throat and alternating hot and cold sensations. Menopausal hot flushes are intermittent periods of heat effusion with vexation that can occur with a periodicity matching the *Xiǎo chái hú tāng* pattern's alternating chills and feverishness. One of *Xiǎo chái hú tāng*'s identifying features is its application for patients with a **depressive** psychological state, accompanied by reluctance to speak, poor appetite, low sex drive and neck and shoulder tension.

- *Tiān wáng bǔ xīn dān* (Heavenly Emperor's Tonify the Heart Pill) calms the *shén*, nourishes heart blood, supplements liver and kidney *yīn* and harmonizes the heart-*shén* and kidney-*zhì*. With the appropriate clinical manifestations (signs of heart and kidney *yīn* insufficiency), it is recommended for peri-/**menopausal syndrome, insomnia** and restless sleep, **forgetfulness** and irritability.

- *Xiāo yáo sàn* (Free Wanderer Powder) harmonizes the liver and spleen to release *qì* constraint. It soothes the liver, strengthens the spleen, regulates *qì* and supplements the blood. With appropriate clinical signs and symptoms (rib-side, chest or abdominal fullness and distending pain, worse with stress, fine wiry pulse), *Xiāo yáo sàn* may be applied in cases of peri-/ **menopausal syndrome, depression, insomnia, anxiety,** poor appetite, **menstrual disorders,** fatigue, irritability, despondency, pent-up frustration.

- Where the *Xiāo yáo sàn qì* constraint pattern transforms into fire, substitute *Jiā wèi xiāo yáo sàn.*

- *Bā wèi shèn qì wán* (Eight Ingredients Kidney *Qì* Pills) warms and strengthens kidney *yáng*. With the appropriate clinical manifestations, it is recommended for peri-/**menopausal syndrome, depression,** somnolence, senile **dementia,** senile itching, **forgetfulness,** hysterical paralysis and **scanty menses**.

- *Suān zǎo rén tāng* (Spiny Jujube Decoction), for *shén–hún* disharmony due to depleted liver and heart *yīn*-blood, is discussed in the next section on insomnia.

Insomnia

Insomnia is not a disease but an important symptom in TCM psychology. Insomnia refers broadly to any form of disturbed sleep or inability to sleep, including dream-disturbed and restless sleep. Disturbed sleeping patterns are common features in all forms of 神志病 *shén zhì bìng*. Chinese medicine has developed various strategies and formulas to address the illness patterns and patho-mechanisms that can affect the *shén*'s ability to settle at night.

One of the few herbal formulas recorded in the *Inner Canon* (*c.* 100 BCE) is for insomnia. 'Pinellia and Millet Decoction' (半夏秫米汤 *Bàn xià shú mǐ tāng*), from the *Divine Pivot* Treatise 71, is designed to address disturbed sleep with palpitations due to **phlegm dampness obstructing the stomach** *qì* and the middle *jiāo*'s ascending–descending *qì* dynamic.

Bàn xià shú mǐ tāng (Pinellia and Millet Decoction):

Zhi ban xia (prepared Rhizoma Pinelliae)   40g

Shu mi (Fructus Setariae/Fructus Sorgum)   50g

The medicinals' respective acrid-warm and sweet-cool natures transform phlegm and restore the *qì* dynamic. Together they clear away turbidity, harmonize the stomach and middle *jiāo* to release constraint when the *zàng shén* are affected by mental–emotional factors.

With appropriate presenting manifestations (lethargy, poor appetite, belching and bitter taste, edema, excessive sputum, nausea, pale tongue), the formula may be used for cases of sleepiness with **insomnia** and restlessness, heavy head, blurred vision, chest oppression.

The *Bàn xià shú mǐ tāng* disharmony is sometimes described as a *yáng* heel vessel[162] vacuity pattern causing *yíng–wèi* disharmony and a failure of the *wèi* defense to move internally at night. By harmonizing the *qì* dynamic, the formula restores the inter-penetrating movements and transformations of *yīn* and *yáng*, which in turn quietens the *shén* and allows it to settle.

According to TCM, we are able to sleep peacefully at night when the *shén* and *hún* settle in the heart and liver *zàng*. Sleeplessness, disturbed sleep, nightmares and excess dreaming occur if they fail to do this. In some cases, the patient is able to remember their dreams clearly when they wake. The patient with a restless *shén* can remember their dreams because the heart-*shén*'s governing role oversees information perception and storage. When the *hún* especially is failing to settle, the patient cannot remember their dreams because the *hún* alone cannot process and remember. In many cases, both the *shén* and *hún* will require 'settling' treatment strategies, but when the patient cannot remember their dreams, more emphasis may be given to calming the *hún*.

The heart-*shén* and liver-*hún* are easily agitated by pathogenic fire and phlegm fire repletion illness states. Depletion states can also cause disturbed sleep. Depleted *yīn* patterns are common because insufficiency of *yīn*-blood at night prevents the *shén* and *hún* from settling peacefully. In addition, the depleted *yīn* tends to produce empty heat that harasses the *shén* and *hún*, leading to restlessness with feelings of vexation, agitation and depression.

For *yīn* depletion illness patterns, the following three formulas address heart and liver (*shén–hún*), heart and lung (*shén–pò*) and heart and kidney (*shén–zhì*) disharmonies. The first is another of the *Golden*

---

162 The *yáng* heel vessel (阳跷脉 *yáng qiào mài*) is one of the eight extraordinary channels

Cabinet's 'Depletion Taxation' formulas, the 'Spiny Jujube Decoction' (酸枣仁汤 *Suān zǎo rén tāng*).

[Line 6.17] For depletion taxation with empty heat, agitation and inability to sleep, *Suān zǎo rén tāng* governs.

Suān zǎo rén tāng (Spiny Jujube Decoction)

Suan zao ren (Semen Ziziphi Spinosi)	18g
Zhi mu (Rhizoma Anemarrhenae)	10g
Fu ling (Sclerotium Poriae Cocos)	12g
Chuan xiong (Rhizoma Chuanxiong)	9g
Gan cao (Radix Glycyrrhizae)	6g

The formula addresses **shén–hún disharmony** due to depleted liver *yīn*-blood. It nourishes *yīn*-blood, regulates liver *qì* and blood, clears heat and eliminates vexation, actions that quieten and harmonize the heart-*shén* and liver-*hún*.

With the appropriate clinical manifestations, it is recommended for **insomnia, sleepwalking**, palpitations, bi-polar, **anxiety** and panic disorders, **psychosis**, **forgetfulness**, peri-/**menopausal syndrome**, fatigue, sleepiness.

Suān zǎo rén tāng is frequently used for the treatment of insomnia. The formula is for patients with **insufficient liver *yīn*-blood** who are unable to fall asleep when they lie down at night due to empty heat harassing the interior and causing vexation. Vexation is a feeling of unease, agitation and listlessness in the heart, accompanied by disturbed sleep or sleeplessness. The *Suān zǎo rén tāng* patient tends to be easily frightened, restless and absent-minded.

Suān zǎo rén tāng is suitable for *shén–hún* disharmony due to *yīn*-blood vacuity, and for the other two types of *shén* disharmonies due to depleted *yīn*, recommended formulas include:

- ***Bǎi hé zhī mǔ tāng*** for *shén–pò* disharmony and heart and lung *yīn* deficiency illness patterns.

- ***Tiān wáng bǔ xīn dān*** for depleted *yīn* states affecting the heart-*shén*, liver-*hún* and kidney-*zhì*.

As well as *Suān zǎo rén tāng*, some of the other *Golden Cabinet* formulas for depletion wasting conditions can be considered for cases with severe depletions affecting the middle *jiāo*, *qì*, blood, *yīn* and *yáng*.

- For example, and with appropriate presenting signs and symptoms, **Xiǎo jiàn zhōng tāng** (Minor Center-Fortifying Decoction) may be used in the treatment of insomnia patients with depression and chronic gastritis. The formula warms and strengthens the spleen and stomach, relieves pain, nourishes the *qì* and blood and harmonizes *yīn* and *yáng*.

For less severe depletions, two more formulas may be considered to nourish the *qì*, blood and *zàng shén*:

- **Gān mài dà zǎo tāng**, which gently nourishes and regulates the five *zàng shén*.

- **Guī pí tāng**, which strengthens and nourishes the *qì*–blood of the spleen and heart and calms the *shén*.

Heart *qì* vacuity insomnia patients will present with sleeplessness, or frequent waking; they are fearful and easily startled, frightened and unsettled by minor things. We introduced 'Settle the Emotions Pill' (定志丸 *Dìng zhì wán*) and 'Calm the Shen and Settle the Mind Pill' (安神定志丸 *Ān shén dìng zhì wán*) above in connection with the visceral agitation illness category. **Dìng zhì wán** is recommended for heart *qì* vacuity, and **Ān shén dìng zhì wán** for dual vacuity of the heart and gallbladder *qì*, a state that may be due to shock or fright.

Dìng zhì wán (Settle the Emotions Pill)

***Ān shén dìng zhì wán*
(Calm the *Shén* and Settle the Emotions Pill)**

Ren shen (Radix Ginseng)	9g
Fu ling (Sclerotium Poriae Cocos)	9g (*15g)
Shi chang pu (Rhizoma Acori Tatarinowii)	6g (*15g)
Yuan zhi (Radix Polygalae)	6g (*15g)
**Fu shen* (Poria Pararadicis)	15g
**Long chi* (Dens Draconis)	15g

Suan zao ren (Semen Zizyphi Spinosae)	15g
Ye jiao teng (Caulis Polygoni Multiflori)	15g
Mu li (Concha Ostreae)	20g
Zhu sha (Cinnabaris)^	5g

Dìng zhì wán strengthens the heart *qì*, resolves turbid phlegm and settles the *shén*. With the addition of the medicinals * above, *Ān shén dìng zhì wán* strengthens both the heart and gallbladder *qì*, supplements *yīn*-blood, and more strongly pacifies the *shén*.

With the appropriate clinical manifestations (fatigue, pale tongue, a wiry and forceless pulse), these formulas are recommended for **insomnia**, nightmares, **forgetfulness**, confusion, **anxiety** and **panic** attacks, obsessive-compulsive disorder (OCD), **depression** (including postpartum depression), **mania** and PMS.

(^ Prohibited substance)

Modifications:

- Substitute *Long chi* or *Zhen zhu* for *Zhu sha*^

Wáng Qīngrèn's *Correcting the Errors in the Forest of Medicine*[163] (1830) drew attention to the role of blood stasis in chronic diseases, including stubborn insomnia. Blood moving formulas such as 'Drive Out Stasis in the Mansion of Blood Decoction' (血府逐瘀汤 *Xuè fǔ zhú yū tāng*) may be applied in cases of heart blood stasis or static blood in the upper *jiāo* and diaphragm area. Static blood conditions post-trauma may be a feature of the patient's medical history.

Xuè fǔ zhú yū tāng
(Drive Out Stasis in the Mansion of Blood Decoction)

Tao ren (Semen Persicae)	12g
Hong hua (Flos Carthami)	9g
Dang gui (Radix Angelicae Sinensis)	9g
Sheng di huang (Radix Rehmanniae)	9g
Chuan xiong (Radix Chuanxiong)	4.5g
Chi shao (Radix Paeoniae Rubra)	6g

163 王清任 Wáng Qīngrèn (1768–1831), 《医林改错》 *Yī lín gǎi cuò*

Zhi ke (Fructus Aurantii)	6g
Chai hu (Radix Bupleuri)	3g
Gan cao (Radix Glycyrrhizae)	6g
Jie geng (Radix Platycodi)	4.5g
Niu xi (Radix Achyranthis)	9g

The formula moves the blood, smooths liver *qì* and unblocks the channels to dispel blood stasis and relieve pain.

With appropriate clinical manifestations (chronic strong fixed stabbing pain, dark complexion, dark/purplish lips, dark red/purple tongue body or spots, choppy pulse), the formula may be used for cases of **insomnia** including stubborn insomnia with restless sleep and dreaming, palpitations, **depression**, mood swings, peri-/**menopausal syndrome**, anger, dizziness, tinnitus, **forgetfulness**, **psychosis** and schizophrenia, post-head-trauma or cerebral vascular accident (post-CVA), post-traumatic stress disorder (PTSD), PMS, dysmenorrhea and endometriosis.

Modifications:

- *Qì* vacuity, – *Chai hu* and *Chuan xiong* and + *Huang qi* and *Dang shén*

- Insufficiency of *yìn*, – *Chai hu* and *Chuan xiong* and + *Gou qi zi* and *Shan zhu yu*

- Blood depletion, – *Chai hu* and *Chuan xiong* and + *Shu di huang* and *Ye jiao teng*

When the *yù zhēng*-constraint pattern is the primary illness pattern in cases of insomnia and restless sleep, it may be appropriate to prescribe:

- **Bàn xià hòu pǔ tāng**, where liver *qì* constraint combines with phlegm dampness accumulations causing throat disorders

or

- **Xiāo yáo sàn** for liver constraint with depleted spleen *qì* and blood

or

- **Jiā wèi xiāo yáo sàn** in cases of constraint transforming into fire.

Constraint transforming into fire is an example of repletion heat states causing insomnia. Representative formulas for other forms of **repletion fire and phlegm heat** illness patterns that cause insomnia include *Chái hú jiā lóng gǔ mǔ lì tāng* and *Wēn dǎn tāng*, two formulas that may also be considered for more severe *shén zhì bìng* such as psychosis.

Psychosis

Psychosis is a severe form of *shén zhì bìng* where the patient is unable to know what is real and what is not. Symptoms therefore include auditory, olfactory, visual and/or tactile hallucinations. Other typical manifestations are disorganized and inappropriate behavior, mania, delirium, disturbed sleep, confused thinking, withdrawal, lassitude, lack of motivation and difficulty engaging with people and daily life. The most common form of psychosis— schizophrenia—often occurs with additional mental–emotional health problems such as anxiety, depressive or substance use disorders.

Yáng type psychosis (狂 *kuáng*) is characterized by mania, delusions, paranoia, hallucinations and incoherent speech. Patients display bizarre behaviors such as talking with imaginary people, attacking others, strange repetitious movements, speech or actions. *Yīn*-type psychosis (癲 *diān*) is characterized by symptoms of withdrawal, reluctance to speak and decreased general awareness. The patient's eyes and facial expression are dull, their thinking and responses are slow.

The treatment of severe *shén zhì bìng* is likely to require aggressive methods such as purgation to expel pathogenic factors, reflecting the ancient belief of evil spirits possessing the patient. The 'Major Bupleurum Decoction' (大柴胡汤 *Dà chái hú tāng*), from Zhāng Zhòngjǐng's *Golden Cabinet* (Chapter 10), is one example of this approach.

Dà chái hú tāng (Major Bupleurum Decoction)

Chai hu (Radix Bupleuri)	24g
Huang qin (Radix Scutellariae)	9g
Bai shao (Radix Paeoniae Alba)	9g
Zhi shi (Fructus Aurantii Immaturus)	9g
Da huang (Radix et Rhizoma Rhei)	6g

Zhi ban xia (prepared Radix Pinelliae)	24g
Sheng jiang (Rhizoma Zingeberis Recens)	15g
Da zao (Fructus Jujubae)	12 pieces

The formula harmonizes the *shǎoyáng*, purges **internal heat accumulation**, drains liver and gallbladder fire, and has a sedating effect.

With appropriate presenting manifestations (fullness and pain below the heart, rib-side fullness with discomfort or pain, alternating sensations of cold/heat, vexation, bitter taste, nausea and vomiting, constipation or foul diarrhoea, asthmatic breathing, yellow tongue coat, sunken wiry forceful pulse), the formula may be used for cases of **psychosis**, schizophrenia, **mania** and mental instability, **depression** with restlessness and despondency, **insomnia**, diminished hearing or eyesight, **dementia** and Alzheimer's disease (in patients with a strong, robust body type).

Modifications:

- Phlegm, + *Yu jin* and *Ming fan*

- Blood stasis, + *Tao ren* and *Gui zhi*

- Manic behavior (liver fire), + *Zhi zi, Mu dan pi, Qing dai, Mang xiao*

To address a complex repletion/depletion pattern featuring **liver–gallbladder constraint** with heat affecting the heart-*shén*, Zhāng Zhòngjǐng recommends 'Bupleurum plus Dragon Bone and Oyster Shell Decoction' (柴胡加龙骨牡蛎汤 *Chái hú jiā lóng gǔ mǔ lì tāng*). The formula is designed to treat thoracic fullness, vexation and terror, and later physicians applied it to cases of mania, feeling frightened, Parkinsonism and epilepsy. The patient's signs and symptoms are likely to have arisen after an episode of drastic emotional stress, for example in some cases of post-traumatic stress disorder (PTSD).

Chái hú jiā lóng gǔ mǔ lì tāng
(Bupleurum plus Dragon Bone and Oyster Shell Decoction)

Chai hu (Radix Bupleuri)	12g
Huang qin (Radix Scutellariae)	4g
Zhi ban xia (prepared Radix Pinelliae)	9g
Ren shen (Radix Ginseng)	5g
Sheng jiang (Rhizoma Zingeberis Recens)	5g
Gui zhi (Ramulus Cinnamomi)	5g
Fu ling (Sclerotium Poriae Cocos)	5g
Long gu (Fossilia Ossis Mastodi)	5g
Mu li (Concha Ostreae)	5g
Da huang (Radix et Rhizoma Rhei) (added near the end)	6g
Da zao (Fructus Jujubae)	6 pieces
Dai zhe shi (Haematitum)^	1g

The formula sedates and settles the *shén*, clears heat and relieves constraint, resolves phlegm dampness and restores the *qì* dynamic.

With appropriate clinical manifestations (chest oppression and fullness, vexation, fright, irritability, restlessness, palpitations, emotional instability, a heavy sinking feeling in the body, red tongue), the formula may be used for cases of delirious speech, **psychosis**, schizophrenia, disordered consciousness and cognition, **mania**, agitation, phobias, **fearfulness** and overreacting to stimulus, overly worried and tending to obsessiveness, PTSD, **depression** and **anxiety** disorders, **menopausal syndrome**, vivid dreams, **insomnia**, inhibited urination, digestive problems, **epilepsy**, hypertension, Parkinson's disease, **dementia**, Alzheimer's disease.

In children (with strong constitution and dry stool): brain dysfunction causing paralysis or delayed development, hyperactivity disorders, sleepwalking.

(^ Restricted substance)

Modifications:

- Insomnia and headache, + *Chuan xiong, Suan zao ren, Gan cao* and *Zhi mu*

When phlegm heat pathogenic factors disturb the *shén*, they obstruct the heart-*shén* aperture and the other sensory openings. They disrupt cognition, mood and perceptions and severely disturb the patient's inner world and their ability to manage their outer world. Signs and symptoms indicating phlegm heat will include gnawing hunger with nausea and slight thirst, a bitter taste in the mouth, reflux and indigestion. The tongue coating will be yellow and greasy, and the pulse rapid and slippery.

For psychological problems presenting with phlegm heat illness patterns, including **phelgm heat obstructing the heart–*shén* aperture**, the representative formula is 'Warm the Gallbladder Decoction' (温胆 汤 *Wēn dǎn tāng*). The formula is from Chén Yán's *Discussion of Illnesses, Patterns, and Formulas Related to the Unification of the Three Aetiologies*[164] (1173).

Wēn dǎn tāng (Warm the Gallbladder Decoction)

Zhu ru (Caulis Bambusae in Taeniis)	6g
Zhi shi (Fructus Immaturus Citri Urantii)	6g
Ban xia (Rhizoma Pinelliae Ternatae)	6g
Chen pi (Pericarpium Citri Reticulatae)	9g
Fu ling (Sclerotium Poriae Cocos)	4.5g
Gan cao (Radix Glycyrrhizae Uralensis)	3g
Sheng jiang (Rhizoma Zingiberis Officinalis Recens)	3–6g
Da zao (Fructus Zizyphi Jujubae)	3 pieces

The formula dissolves phlegm heat, clears the gallbladder, relieves constraint and regulates the stomach.

With appropriate signs and symptoms, the formula can be applied in cases of heart and gallbladder susceptibility to fright, severe and stubborn **insomnia**, vivid dreaming and nightmares, epilepsy, **psychosis**, schizophrenia and **hallucinations**, senile **dementia**, timidity, easily startled, **depression**, obsessive-compulsive disorders, PTSD, bi-polar, panic and **anxiety** disorders, fearfulness, phobias, **menopausal syndrome**, palpitations, restlessness, stuffy feeling in the chest, dizziness, tinnitus and deafness.

---

164 《三因极一病证方论》 *Sān yīn jí yī bìng zhèng fāng lùn*

Modifications:

- Strong heat, + *Huang lian* = ***Huāng lián wēn dǎn tāng***

Pathological products (phlegm dampness and static blood) are a common complication, or sometimes a prominent feature, of *shén zhì bìng* patterns, and **static blood** is often accompanied by **phlegm obstruction**. 'Awaken from the Nightmare of Madness Decoction' (癫狂梦醒汤 *Diān kuáng mèng xǐng tāng*) is specifically for psychotic disorders due to static blood with phlegm obstruction. *Diān kuáng mèng xǐng tāng* is from the static blood formula family developed by Wáng Qīngrèn and recorded in his *Correcting the Errors in the Forrest of Medicine* (1830).

Diān kuáng mèng xǐng tāng
(Awaken from the Nightmare of Madness Decoction)

Tao ren (Semen Persicae)	24g
Chai hu (Radix Bupleuri)	9g
Xiang fu (Rhizoma Cyperi)	6g
Mu tong (Caulis Akebiae)	6g
Chi shao (Radix Paeoniae Rubra)	9g
Zhi ban xia (Rhizoma Pinelliae Preparatum)	6g
Da fu pi (Pericarpium Arecae)	9g
Qing pi (Pericarpium Citri Reticulatae Viride)	6g
Chen pi (Pericarpium Citri Reticulatae)	9g
Sang bai pi (Cortex Mori)	9g
Zi su zi (Fructus Perillae)	12g
Gan cao (Radix Glycyrrhizae)	6g

The formula transforms blood stasis, moves blood and stagnant *qì*, transforms phlegm and harmonizes the middle *jiāo*.

With appropriate presenting manifestations (dark complexion, purple tongue body or spots with a white coat, choppy pulse), the formula may be used for cases of anger, **psychosis** and schizophrenia, bi-polar disorder, **depression**, incessant crying, incoherent speech, **mania**, agitation, restlessness.

In some psychosis cases, or in some stages in the treatment of psychosis, it will be more appropriate to, for example:

- gently harmonize the emotions and the *qì* of the five *zàng shén*:

  - ***Gān mài dà zǎo tāng*** + *Long gu* and *Mu li*
  or

  - ***Gān mài dà zǎo tāng*** + ***Bǎi hé gù jīn tāng*** (Lily Bulb Preserve the Metal Decoction) settles the heart-*shén*, liver-*hún* and lung-*pò*, harmonizes the middle *qì* and relaxes tension

- restore the *qì* dynamic:

  - ***Bēn tún tāng*** soothes the liver, harmonizes the stomach, moves and nourishes the blood, relaxes tension and clears heat to relieve the heart-*shén*

- release constraint and restore correct movement of *qì*:

  - ***Bàn xià hòu pǔ tāng*** transforms phlegm, benefits the stomach and strengthens the spleen.

Anxiety

Under the broad heading of anxiety, Western psychology distinguishes a number of different diseases, such as generalized anxiety, panic and phobia disorders, post-traumatic stress and obsessive-compulsive disorders (PTSD and OCD). Patients diagnosed with any of these tend to be overly tense, nervous and fearful. Patients with fearfulness, and those diagnosed with anxiety and panic disorders, are likely to also present with sleep disturbances. During acute episodes such as panic attacks, there may be breathing difficulties, palpitations, dizziness, nausea, chest and abdominal discomfort.

Chinese medicine treatments for anxiety commonly employ medicinals that 'quieten the *shén*,' such as *Long gu* and *Mu li. Guì zhī jiā lóng gǔ mǔ lì tāng* (Cinnamon Twig plus Dragon Bone and Oyster Shell Decoction) is an example.

- From the *Golden Cabinet* Chapter 6 (see 'depletion taxation'), ***Guì zhī jiā lóng gǔ mǔ lì tāng*** treats a state whereby weakened *yīn* essence draining away below is unable to restrain depleted *yáng* floating above, a condition due to excess sex, loss of blood, or other forms of exhaustion from overwork or illness. In the *Golden Cabinet*, the formula secures the essence and **restores and harmonizes the *yīn* and *yáng*.** TCM textbooks identify the pattern as **liver–kidney *yáng* vacuity cold**.

- Both *Guì zhī jiā lóng gǔ mǔ lì tāng*, and ***Chái hú jiā lóng gǔ mǔ lì tāng*** (Bupleurum plus Dragon Bone and Oyster Shell Decoction, discussed in the previous section on 'Psychosis') treat insomnia, fearfulness and hypersensitivity. While *Guì zhī jiā lóng gǔ mǔ lì tāng* is indicated for depleted *jīng*-essence with *yáng* vacuity cold patterns, *Chái hú jiā lóng gǔ mǔ lì tāng* addresses **repletion heat from liver–gallbladder *qì* constraint with dampness accumulation** affecting the *shén*.

'Fried Liquorice Decoction' (炙甘草汤 *Zhì gān cǎo tāng*) is an appended formula from the *Golden Cabinet* Chapter 6 (Line 6.18). In this form of depletion taxation, the blood, *qì*, *yīn* and *yáng* are severely depleted. *Yáng* vacuity sweating is unable to secure the defense *qì* on the body surface and consequently *yīn*-fluids cannot be guarded internally. Because the *qì* and blood are in a weakened state, they cannot circulate effectively and the heart *qì* is devitalized through lack of nourishment. The formula is also known as 'Restore the Pulse Decoction,' and may be applied in cases of **heart *qì* deficiency**, or **general *qì*-blood-*yīn* deficiency** due to excess worry and emotions injuring the heart and spleen.

Zhì gān cǎo tāng (Fried Liquorice Decoction)	
Zhi gan cao (prepared Radix Glycyrrhizae)	12g
Gui zhi (Ramulus Cinnamomi)	9g
Sheng jiang (Rhizoma Zingeberis Recens)	9g
Mai men dong (Radix Ophiopogonis)	9g
Huo ma ren (Semen Cannabis)	9g
Ren shen (Radix Ginseng)	6g
E jiao (Asini Corii Colla)	6g
Da zao (Fructus Jujubae)	30 pieces
Sheng di huang (Radix Rehmanniae)	48g

The formula strengthens the *qì*, nourishes the blood, supplements the *yīn* and restores the pulse.

With appropriate clinical manifestations (palpitations with anxiety, dry mouth and throat, emaciation, pale shiny tongue, irregular slow thin faint pulse), the formula may be used for cases of **anxiety**, restlessness, **insomnia**, irritability, **forgetfulness**, shortness of breath.

Modifications:

- Insomnia, – *Huo ma ren* and + *Suan zao ren*

- Poor concentration and memory, + *Shi chang pu*

For **yáng qì vacuity**, the 'True Warrior Decoction' (真武汤 *Zhēn wǔ tāng*) from Zhāng Zhòngjǐng's *On Cold Damage* is designed to strengthen the kidney, spleen and heart *yáng*, and drain untransformed fluids by urination. When the *yáng qì* is deficient, pathogenic fluids ('water *qì*') may be used for cases of consequently obstructed urinary functions. They can spill into the flesh and skin causing edema, and may cause water *qì* flooding in the upper *jiāo* that intimidates the heart.

Zhēn wǔ tāng (True Warrior Decoction)

Pao fu zi (prepared Radix Aconiti Lateralis)	9g
Bai zhu (Rhizoma Atractylodis Macrocephalae)	6g
Fu ling (Sclerotium Poriae Cocos)	9g
Sheng jiang (Rhizoma Zingiberis Recens)	9g
Bai shao (Radix Paeoniae Alba)	9g

The formula strengthens the *yáng* and promotes urination.

With appropriate clinical manifestations (abdominal pain worse with cold, heavy aching cold limbs, heavy head, swollen tongue with white wet fur, deep forceless pulse), the formula may be used for mental–emotional disorders, palpitations with chest discomfort, severe fatigue, **anxiety**, dizziness and feeling unstable, **insomnia**, poor memory, **forgetfulness**, dimmed vision, husky voice.

Depending on specific presentations, many of the previous formulas may apply to anxiety disorders. Pattern differentiation to identify *qì*, *yīn* and blood depletion patterns, phlegm dampness obstruction, fire or phlegm fire repletion patterns for example, will be needed to focus the treatment strategy and address the patient's underlying body state.

- **Gān mài dà zǎo tāng** to nourish and harmonize all the *zàng qì* and *shén*.

- **Guī pí tāng** to supplement the *qì* and blood of the heart and spleen.

- **Dìng zhì wán/Ān shén dìng zhì wán** strengthens heart and gallbladder *qì* depletion (including that due to shock or fright).

- **Xiāo yáo sàn** (or **Jiā wèi xiāo yáo sàn**) for liver *qì* constraint (or *qì* constraint transforming into fire) disturbing the *shén*.

- **Bàn xià hòu pǔ tāng** for liver *qì* constraint with phlegm accumulation (plum pit *qì*).

- **Suān zǎo rén tāng** nourishes heart and liver *yīn*-blood, and clears empty heat to settle the *shén*.

- **Tiān wáng bǔ xīn dān** supplements heart and kidney *yīn*, clears empty heat to calm the *shén*.

- **Wēn dǎn tāng** clears and resolves liver-gallbladder phlegm fire disturbing the *shén*.

- **Bēn tún tāng** nourishes and moves the blood, soothes the liver, harmonizes the stomach and restores *qì* descending.

Dementia

Forgetfulness and memory loss can occur at any time, although they are most often associated with aging. Under this heading, we include a number of mental–physical infirmities, behavioral and cognitive symptoms and diseases that tend to occur in later life. Neurocognitive disorders such as Alzheimer's disease and vascular dementia are more common in older patients and defined by declining memory and loss of cognitive function. Vascular dementia patients typically have a history of cerebral infarctions and hypertension, and both kinds of patients are likely to suffer the behavioral and psychological symptoms of dementia, including agitation and depression.

Although Chinese medicine theory would suggest the likelihood of depletion patterns in older patients (depletions of *qì*, blood, *yīn*, *yáng* or *jīng*-essence or the sea of marrow), clinical practice demonstrates the importance of clearing away pathogenic factors (邪气 *xié qì*), supporting correct *qì* (正气 *zhèng qì*) and regulating *qì* functions. Classical and contemporary Chinese medicine treatments also tend to support the *yīn*-blood and *yáng-qì* of the heart, spleen and kidney *zàng shén*, although not only these. Important strategies include removing static blood, dissolving phlegm, opening the apertures, strengthening *qì*, nourishing the blood and harmonizing functional relationships.

To dispel pathogenic factors, several strategies may be considered. When turbid phlegm dampness obstructs the apertures, or in other words, when the diagnosis is **'phlegm misting the heart,'** 'Cleanse the Heart Decoction' (洗心汤 *Xǐ xīn tāng*) is recommended.

Xǐ xīn tāng (Cleanse the Heart Decoction)

Ren shen (Radix Genseng)	12g
Suan zao ren (Semen Zizyphi Spinosae)	12g
Fu shen (Poria Pararadicis)	12g
Zhi ban xia (prepared Rhizoma Pinelliae)	9g
Chen pi (Pericarpium Citri Reticulatae)	6g
Shen qu (Massa Medicata Fermentata)	6g
Zhi fu zi (prepared Radix Aconiti Lateralis)	3g
Shi chang pu (Rhizoma Acori Tatarinowii)	9g
Gan cao (Radix Glyyrrhizae)	6g

The formula strengthens the spleen, resolves phlegm, arouses the brain, opens the apertures.

With appropriate clinical manifestations (edema, weakness, fatigue, swollen pale tongue with white slimy coat, soggy and slippery pulse), the formula may be used for **dementia**, mental **confusion** and confused speech, **forgetfulness**, mood swings, hypersomnia, Alzheimer's disease.

If diagnosis finds that **phlegm heat** pathogenic products **obstruct the heart–*shén* aperture**, we drain heat and resolve phlegm using, for example, 'Flush the Phlegm Decoction' (荡痰汤 *Dàng tán tāng*).

Dàng tán tāng (Flush the Phlegm Decoction)

Dai zhe shi (Haematitum)^   60g

Zhi ban xia (Rhizoma Pinelliae Preparatum) 9g

Da huang (Radix et Rhizoma Rhei)   30g

Mang xiao (Natrii Sulfas)   18g

Yu jin (Radix Curcumae)   9g

The formula drains heat and dissolves phlegm.

With appropriate clinical manifestations (feverish, dry stools, difficult breathing, nausea, scarlet tongue with yellow greasy tongue coat, rapid slippery pulse), the formula may be applied in cases of **mania**, **psychosis**, OCD, bi-polar disorder, **anxiety**, **dementia**, forgetfulness, **depression**, despondency

(^ Restricted substance)

Wáng Qīngrèn's static blood formulas equip us with another important strategy for patients with forgetfulness, memory loss and dementia. *Xuè fǔ zhú yū tāng* is appropriate for the static heart blood and liver *qì* constraint illness pattern (discussed in the 'Insomnia' section).

More specifically for **static blood obstructing the brain collaterals**, 'Open the Apertures and Quicken the Blood Decoction' (通窍活血汤 *Tōng qiào huó xuè tāng*) is recommended. Wáng Qīngrèn advises that this formula unblocks all the small vessels and openings throughout the body, not only the sensory apertures in the head.

Tōng qiào huó xuè tāng (Open the Apertures and Quicken the Blood Decoction)

Tao ren (Semen Persicae)   9g

Hong hua (Flos Carthami)   9g

Chuan xiong (Radix Chuanxiong)   3g

Chi shao (Radix Paeoniae Rubra)   3g

Cong bai (Bulbus Allii Fistulosi)   3g

Da zao (Fructus Jujubae)   7 pieces

Sheng jiang (Rhizoma Zingiberis Recens)   9g

She xiang (Moschus)^   0.15g

The formula activates blood and dispels stasis, opens the apertures and blood vessels.

With appropriate clinical manifestations (stabbing, chronic, strong, fixed pain in the head, face or upper body, dark complexion, dark around the eyes or nose, dark/purplish lips, dark tongue body or purplish spots, choppy pulse), the formula may be used for patients with a history of epidural hemorrhage or cerebrovascular accident (CVA), and for cases of dimmed eyesight, hearing loss, deafness, dizziness, unclear speech, **dementia**, confusion, **depression**, vexation, restlessness, agitation, **insomnia** and sleepiness.

(^ CITES Endangered species)

Modifications:

- Substitute *Yu jin* (6g) for *She xiang^*

- To purge repletion heat with static blood, replace with ***Táo hé chéng qì tāng*** (for strong patients, and robust body type)

- For static blood with blood deficiency, *Chi shao, Cong bai, Sheng jiang, Yu jin* and + *Shu di huang, Bai shao* and *Dang gui* = ***Táo hóng sì wù tāng***

Once pathogenic factors have been resolved and eliminated, deficiency patterns may need to be addressed. Common deficiency illness patterns causing forgetfulness and senile dementia affect the *yīn, yáng*, blood and *qì* of the five *zàng*. Depleted *jīng*-essence affecting kidney-*zhì* functions and relationships is also common. The mansion of essence, the brain, is the material basis of *shén míng* clarity and intelligence, and Zhāng Jièbīn's (1563–1640) 'Seven Blessings Decoction' (七福汤 *Qī fú tāng*) **nourishes heart blood, strengthens spleen *qì* and benefits the brain.**

***Qī fú tāng* (Seven Blessings Decoction)**	
Ren shen (Radix Ginseng)	15g
Shu di (prepared Radix Rehmanniae)	25g
Suan zao ren (Fructus Zizyphi Spinosae)	15g
Dang gui (Radix Angelicae Sinensis)	20g
Bai zhu (Rhizoma Atractylodis Macrocephalae)	15g

Yuan zhi (Radix Polygalae)	15g
Da zao (Fructus Ziziphus Jujube)	4 pieces
Zhi gan cao (Radix Glycyrrhizae)	5g

The formula boosts *qì* and blood movement, strengthens the heart, spleen, kidney, brain and the *yáng qì*, and calms the *shén*.

With appropriate clinical manifestations (sallow complexion, fatigue, low sperm count, poor appetite, pale tongue, forceless pulse), the formula may be used for cases of **dementia**, impotence, **forgetfulness**, **anxiety** and panic attacks, palpitations, **insomnia** and dream-disturbed sleep.

Other formulas commonly prescribed for dementia and Alzheimer's disease address the following presentations and illness patterns:

- *Tiān wáng bǔ xīn dān* for heart and kidney *yīn* vacuity.

- *Zhēn wǔ tāng* for insufficiency of the kidney *yáng*, with spleen and heart *yáng* vacuity.

- *Guī pí tāng* for insufficiency of spleen *qì* and heart blood.

- *Dìng zhì wán* for heart *qì* vacuity.

Chapter 9

Cases

Thinking
Looking at books and forgetting to eat

A scholar read so many books he forgot to eat. One day someone dressed in purple visited him and said: 'You cannot think for too long because it may kill you.' The scholar asked, 'Who are you?' and the person in purple replied, 'I am the God of Grain.' Then the scholar stopped thinking and reading so much, and went back to eating normally.

The above case is from the book *Ancient and Modern Medical Cases*, 'The Seven Emotions: Thinking'[165] (1778).

Notes

Scholars read books attentively and with great concentration. Too much 'thinking knots the *qì*,'[166] and this impairs the spleen's transporting and transforming function. Such people are likely to lose their appetite or have no sense of hunger, and take little food.

The spleen transforms and transports water and food, and the spleen *shén* is sometimes called 谷神 *Gǔ shén*, the 'God of Grain.'

Over-thinking results in no sense of hunger and a poor appetite, and lack of food leads to insufficient grain *qì* (stomach *qì*). The God of Grain came to save the scholar by transforming itself into the image of a person. This was a kind of survival instinct to motivate the scholar to eat regularly. Regular eating continuously reinforces the stomach *qì*.

The *Jīng* ('Classic') states: 'Stomach *qì* maintains life and insufficient stomach *qì* leads to death. Stomach *qì* is also called gu *qì*.'

---

165 《古今医案按 · 七情 · 思》 *Gǔ jīn yī àn àn, Qī qíng: Sī*
166 思则气结 *sī zé qì jié*

Joy

Joy therapy

'Joy therapy' means trying to amuse people to treat their diseases. Liver (wood) repletion illnesses can be treated by applying reducing methods to the heart (fire), its child. While anger leads to *qì* stagnation and hyperactivity, joy slows and relaxes the *qì*. Joy can therefore be used therapeutically to release anger and regulate liver *qì*, and so the disease is treated.

1. Anger and constraint cause illness, joyful playing cures it

The famous doctor Mr. Xu treated a lady who was sick from excess anger. She was bed-ridden and could not even turn over, and no treatment could help her. When he came to visit the patient, Mr. Xu dressed as an old lady holding flowers. He sang, laughed and amused the lady, who watched and laughed with him. Then she was able to turn her body and the problem was cured.

The above case is from *Integrating Ancient and Modern Books*, 'Medical Records: Famous medical cases.'[167]

Notes

The liver governs the sinews and its emotion manifests as anger. Unhappiness leads to liver *qì* stagnation and when triggered by anger, the *qì* ascends. Then the sinews are not properly nourished and the body cannot turn.

When someone suffers from a disorder of the seven emotions, treatments for the physical body do not work. This doctor treated the patient by amusing her, which regulated and smoothed the movement of *qì*, which in turn nourished and relaxed the sinews. Once her sinews were well nourished again, the patient could turn her body and was cured.

Emotional therapy must be practiced in a flexible way. Rather than using sadness to overcome anger, Mr. Xu demonstrated that joy may be used to relax and harmonize the body and mind.

---

167 《古今图书集成 · 医部全录: 医术名流列传》 *Gǔ jīn tú shū jí chéng, Yī bù quán lù: Yī shù míng liú liè zhuàn*

2. Happiness overcomes grief and heartache

A governor in the city of Xi heard that his father had been killed by a robber. The governor wept with grief, and afterwards his heart was aching. For more than one month the pain below his heart worsened. It began to feel like it was growing and forming a mass, as if it were covered by an upside-down cup.

Medicinal substances were not effective. They thought to try warm needling with moxa but the patient couldn't bear it, so they asked for help from the sage Zhāng Cóngzhèng. When the sage came, a shaman was sitting next to the governor raving and talking crazily. The sage then imitated the shaman as a joke to cheer up his patient. The governor could not help laughing, and turned his face to the wall to hide his embarrassment. But in one or two days, the mass he felt below his heart had scattered.

Zhāng Cóngzhèng said that, according to the *Inner Canon*, worry binds the *qì*, and when we are happy, the hundred vessels are relaxed, smooth and harmonized. Thus, it is said: happiness overcomes sadness. This is the *Inner Canon*'s rule of treatment. Why do we need to apply needle and moxa that only cause pain?

The above case is from 'Sadness and Worry Cause Blockages and Accumulations' in the 'Ten Forms and Three Treatments' section of the *Confucians' Duties to Their Parents*[168] by Zhāng Cóngzhèng (1156–1228).

Notes

According to the *Elementary Questions* Treatise 5, worry and sadness damage the lung, and happiness overcomes them. This method is derived from the theory of the five phases, which states that happiness belongs to fire; worry and sadness belong to metal; fire controls metal; therefore, happiness overcomes worry and sadness.

---

168 《儒门事亲 · 十形三疗 · 因忧结块》 *Rú mén shì qīn, Shí xíng sān liáo: Yīn yōu jié kuài*

Fear overcomes excess joy

Too much joy damages the heart

When a scholar received the highest honor in the imperial examination, he returned to his home town. As he passed through Jiangsu, he became ill with a laughing disorder and went to see a famous local doctor, Yuan Tian. The doctor said to him, 'You cannot be helped in any way and you will die in seven days. But if you hurry you will still be able to return home before it is too late.' The scholar felt very concerned and hurried back home, and yet, seven days later he was feeling fine.

His servant then came to him and said, 'The doctor asked me to give you this letter after your return home.' The scholar opened the letter and it read, 'You were too excited after receiving the highest honor in the imperial exam, and excess joy damaged your heart. This cannot be helped by any medication, so I treated you with fear of death. Thus you were cured, and now you are fine.' The scholar felt deeply respectful towards the doctor.

The above case is from *The Whirling Stream of Medicine*, by Xú Dàchūn[169] (1693–1771).

Notes

The *Divine Pivot* '*Běn Shén*' says that too much joy causes the *shén* to spread outwards, with nothing to hold it. Deficient heart *qì* can cause depression, while excessive heart *qì* can cause non-stop laughing. Too much joy damages the heart, causes the *qì* to slacken, and then the *shén* is not held. It spreads out and illness certainly follows. In this case, the scholar's excitement and euphoria had led to madness.

Fear overcomes joy. After being told that his illness was incurable and he would die in seven days, the scholar's fear overcame his elation, just as kidney-water (fear) restrains heart-fire (joy). Thus, he recovered from his emotional disorder.

Isn't it wonderful? Only superior doctors can achieve this!

---

169 《洄溪医书》, 徐大春 *Huí xī yī shū*, Xú Dàchūn

Excess joy causing kuáng-madness

Mr. Fan received a letter and when he read it, he clapped his hands, laughed and said, 'Ooo... Great! I won it!' Then he fell backward clenching his teeth and lost consciousness. An old lady next to him was startled, and she put some water in his mouth. As Mr. Fan came to and got up, he clapped his hands and laughed incessantly: 'Ooo... This is great! I won! I won it!' He ran out of the room, and the postman and neighbors felt scared. Mr. Fan then fell into a pond, struggled out with disarranged hair, muddy hands and his whole body dripping wet. People could not restrain him as he clapped and laughed and walked to the market. Then they realized that Mr. Fan had succeeded in the imperial examination and gone crazy due to the excitement and exhilaration.

The postman said, 'I have an idea but am not sure it will work.' When the other people asked, 'What is your idea?' the postman said, 'Mr. Fan was far too excited, and phlegm came up and blocked his heart. Is he afraid of anyone? What he needs now is to have his face slapped by someone he fears. This person should tell him that the information he received is fake and he has not passed the examination at all. As soon as he is shocked and frightened, he will spit out the sputum and wake up.'

All the other people agreed it sounded like a wonderful idea. Mr. Fan was normally afraid of his father-in-law Mr. Hu, the local butcher. They asked Mr. Hu to confront Mr. Fan in a scary way. He did so and slapped Mr. Fan's face: 'Bloody fool! You did not win it at all!'

The blow caused Mr. Fan to fall to the ground unconscious, and his neighbors came to help him. They massaged his chest and tapped his back for a period of time, then gradually his breathing returned to normal. When he woke up, he had bright eyes and had regained his sanity.

The above case is from the *History of Confucianism*[170] (1749).

---

170 《儒林外史》 *Rú lín wài shǐ*

> **Notes**
>
> Mr. Fan had failed the imperial examinations many times, but after many years of hard study he finally passed. So, he was too excited and the *qì* rushed upwards taking turbid phlegm with it, which blocked his heart aperture. When phlegm covers the aperture, it obstructs and muddles the *shén*. In this way, excess joy caused the madness.
>
> Different emotions can overcome each other and fear can overcome joy. Therefore, since Mr. Fan was most scared of him, Mr. Hu was asked to intervene. After being slapped by this demoniacal man, Mr. Fan's fear overcame his euphoria, his *qì* movement was stabilized and his *shén* was retrieved.

Shén–hún disharmony, *hún* wandering

Evil enters the liver channel, causing dream-disturbed sleep

The mind is unclear, sleep is disturbed by dreams, the *shén* is disturbed and the *hún* wanders. The patient instantly wakes due to any sound, then fails to go back to sleep for the rest of the night. The middle position of their left pulse is full and wiry; therefore, this is not a heart deficiency disorder. The signs and symptoms indicate that the liver channel is caught by evils. Since the *hún* is stored in the liver, it has no place to dwell when the liver suffers from depleted blood. So the *hún* wanders and this manifests as disrupted sleep. People have their own different true understandings about this—please see my prescription.

(*Duan*) *Long chi* (Dens Draconis)	6g
Yuan zhi (Radix Polygalae)	3g
(*Chao*) *Bai shao* (Radix Paeoniae Alba)	9g
Dang gui (Radix Angelicae Sinensis)	3g
Bai zi ren (Semen Platycladi)	3g
(*Bai*) *Fu ling* (Sclerotium Poriae Cocos)	9g
Mai dong (Radix Ophiopogonis)	3g
Ba ji tian (Radix Morindae Officinalis)	3g
Tu si zi (Semen Cuscutae)	3g

(*Chao*) *Suan zao ren* (Semen Zizyphi Spinosae)   6g

Boil in water.

The above is from the 'Palpitations [Fearful Throbbing]' section in the *Nan Ya Tang Medical Cases*[171] (published in 2009 by the People's Army Medical Publishing House, from notes left by 陈修园 Chén Xiūyuán 1753–1823).

Notes

The *Inner Canon* states that the *hún* dwells in the eyes and when we are asleep it is stored in the liver. The liver also stores the blood, and liver blood holds the *hún*; thus, when there is insufficient liver blood, the liver fails to hold the *hún*. When the *hún* is unsettled, the *shén* is not calm, and both the *shén* and the *hún* are disturbed and wander away. Therefore, the patient's body form and mind are not harmonious. Their mind is unclear and they have many dreams while sleeping, the *hún* is disturbed and unsettled, waking up due to any sound and failing to go back to sleep for the whole night.

Long chi and *Yuan zhi* are used to sedate fright and settle the *shén* and *hún*.

Bai shao, Dang gui, Suan zao ren, Bai zi ren, Bai Fu ling (*Fu ling-Poria*, 白 *bái* means the white inner part) and *Mai dong* are used to nourish blood and *yīn*, calm the *shén* and hold the *hún*.

Ba ji tian and *Tu si zi* are added to strengthen the kidney *yáng* and *jīng*-essence, and nourish the *shén*. This follows the principle recorded in the *Elementary Questions* Treatise 3 whereby, 'if the *yáng qì* is firm, it nourishes the *shén*.'

Hún–pò wandering

Nightmares

Mr. Qian suddenly began suffering from nightmares. The nightmares started as soon as he fell asleep and lasted the whole night. While on his travels to a new working position, he met Mr. Hu from Deng Zhou and they talked about his nightmares. Mr. Hu said that he himself used to have the same problem, which frightened him a great deal; but then he

---

171 《南雅堂医案 · 怔忡门》 *Nán yǎ táng yī àn, Zhēng chōng mén*

met a Daoist priest who taught him to wear *Dan sha*[172] in his hair bun. Mr. Hu followed the Daoist's advice and found it worked really well.

Mr. Hu had not had any bad dreams for four or five years, so he believed this was a valuable practice. Mr. Hu then took a small bag from his hair bun and gave it to Mr. Qian, who that night slept soundly with a calm *shén–hún* and no dreams.

Some texts such as the *Genuine Instructions*[173] (1223) record that *Dan sha* helps to prevent attack by external evils. It is true!

The case is from the *Famous Medical Cases*, 'Many Dreams'[174] (1770).

Notes

The heart stores the *shén* and the liver stores the *hún*. The *Divine Pivot* Treatise 8 states that the *hún* is the one who comes and goes with the *shén*. Failure to store either of them results in dream-disturbed sleep and insomnia.

The *Essential Prescriptions of the Golden Cabinet,* Line 11.12 states that: 'A patient with depleted *qì* and blood experiences fear, desires to sleep, dreams of traveling afar, their *jīng*-essence and *shén* are dispersed and separated, and there is unruly wandering of the *hún–pò*.'

The book *Emergency Moxibustion Methods*[175] (1226) recorded that anyone who suffers from nightmares is likely to have a weakened body constitution due to diminished *shén* (神) and *qì* deficiency. This weakened state means that when sleeping, the *shén* cannot be kept within, and the *hún–pò* wanders outwards.

Zhāng Jièbīn said that because the heart stores the *shén*, a tranquil heart results in a clear and peaceful *shén*, and because the *hún* follows the *shén*, a disturbed *shén* upsets the *hún*. Therefore, the treatment principle should be: calm the *shén* to calm the *hún* and then the disorder is resolved.

---

172 Alternate name for 硃砂 *Zhu sha* (Cinnabaris); 丹 *dan* (or 朱 *zhu*) is red in color, and the Chinese believe that it protects from evil

173 《真诰》 *Zhēn gào*, originally authored by 陶弘景 Táo Hóngjǐng (456–536), nowadays is a section of the great compendium of Daoist texts, the 《道藏》 *Dào zàng* (the *Daoist Canon*)

174 《名医类案 · 多梦》 *Míng yī lèi àn, Duō mèng*

175 《备急灸法》 *Bèi jí jiǔ fǎ*

Dan sha enters the heart and kidney to calm and settle the *shén* and treat shock. The *Root Canon*[176] recommends it for nourishing the *jīng shén* and calming the *hún–pò*. *Dan sha* can be made into pills and hung outside the clothes; however, the Daoist priest had cleverly devised a way to place it in the hair bun because the brain is the house of the *yuán shén* (元神). In this way, *Dan sha*'s heavy quality and descending nature calms the *shén* without risking the toxic effects of ingesting it.

Mr. Jiang, the original author of this case, notes that the reasons for dreaming while asleep come from what we have been experiencing and thinking during the day. If we wish to sleep without dreams, we should cultivate stillness and want for nothing during the daytime.

When we are truly able to calm the mind, how can dreams come?

Sleepwalking

Sleepwalking (梦游 *mèng yóu*) occurs during sleep when the *shén, hún, pò, yì* and *zhì* should be stored in their respective *zàng*. Zhāng Zhòngjǐng described its pathogenesis in Chapter 11 of his *Essential Prescriptions of the Golden Cabinet*. There he says that evil crying can upset the *hún* and *pò*, and consume the *qì* and blood. When the heart lacks *qì* and blood, the patient scares easily. After falling asleep, the dreamer travels far away, the *shén* is scattered and the *hún* and *pò* wander frenetically. This scattering of the *shén* with *hún–pò* wandering is regarded as the cause of sleepwalking.

The *Divine Pivot*, '*Běn Shén*' says that the *hún* normally comes and goes with the *shén*. But during sleepwalking, the *hún* fails to settle in the liver or to follow the *shén* lodging in the heart. The liver-*hún* restlessly leaves its place in the liver and controls the sleepwalker's actions instead of the heart-*shén*. The liver opens to the eyes, it nourishes the sinews, which keeps the bones and joints functioning well to facilitate body movement, and the sleepwalker seems able to see well enough to walk, even for long distances, without falling over obstacles. This kind of walking is related to the liver-*hún*.

What the heart is thinking is the *yì*, and when this is kept in the heart for some time it converts into the *zhì*. However, this conscious thought process cannot function properly when the heart-*shén* fails to govern it.

---

176 《本经》 *Běn jīng*, this is another name for the *Shen Nong's Herbal Classic* (Han dynasty)

Therefore, without the heart-*shén*, sleepwalking is non-conscious and sleepwalkers cannot remember what they did in their sleep.

The shén and hún separate, the hún wanders

Mr. Long, a 14-year-old student, came for his first treatment in 1970. Every time he went to sleep, he leapt up from his bed, opened the door, rushed into the field and fell, and was still deeply asleep. Sometimes he walked up to 25 kilometers and sometimes he was injured when he fell. He seemed mentally fine but he complained of restlessness and tinnitus. He knew he had frightening dreams but could not remember walking out of his home. His tongue was red with yellow coating, and the pulse was wiry and rapid.

The treatment method was to clear heart fire to calm the *shén* and subdue the liver to stabilize the *hún*. *Zhū shā ān shén wán* and *Cí zhū wán* were applied. The prescription contained:

Sheng di (Radix Rehmannia)	60g
Huang lian (Rhizoma Coptidis)	18g
Dang gui (Radix Angelicae Sinensis)	30g
Gan cao (Radix Glycyrrhizae)	15g
Duan ci shi (Magnetitum, calcined)^	30g
Jian qu (Massa Medicata Fermentata)	18g

(^ Restricted substance)

The herbs are ground, mixed with honey and made into pills. Nine grams of elutriated *Zhu sha* (aqueous trituration of Cinnabaris) is used to coat the pills, each of which is about the size of a yellow bean. The patient was asked to take 30 pills twice a day, morning and evening. After taking two bags of the prescription, he was cured. (*Jian qu* is another name for *Shen qu*.)

The above case is from the *Journal of Chinese Medicine*, 1981, no. 11.

Notes

This is a typical case of sleepwalking, with the *shén* and *hún* separating and the *hún* wandering. Normally, the heart-*shén* governs all five *zàng shén* and coordinates their respective functions, and the *Divine Pivot* Treatise 8 states that the *hún* comes and goes with the *shén*. It also states that the heart takes charge of perceptions and understanding the outside world, so the heart-*shén* is called the perception *shén* which governs human conscious awareness.

This idea is the same as the Buddhist notion of consciousness which arises through the sensory faculties—the eye, ear, nose, tongue and body—and the awareness. This patient is quite young so his *shén qì* is not yet strong. His red tongue with yellow coating and his wiry and rapid pulse are signs of a heat evil that disturbed his *shén* and separated it from the *hún*. In these conditions, when the liver-*hún* replaces the *shén*'s governance of body–mind activities, sleepwalking can easily happen.

Normally, when we sleep the *shén* settles in the heart and the *hún* in the liver, but when sleepwalking, the *hún* wanders away from the liver. It wanders alone and is not accompanied by the *shén*. The liver opens to the eyes and governs visual functions. It nourishes and governs the sinews and the *Classic* states that the liver thereby maintains the proper functioning of the bones and joints.[177] This means the liver actually has an important role in the body's mobility. In his sleep, this patient jumped up with fright, opened the door and rushed out into the field, and even wandered as far as 25 kilometers away from home. He knew he was having lots of frightening dreams but could not remember them and he stayed deeply asleep even when falling down in the field. This confirms that his sleepwalking was governed by the liver-*hún*. The pattern was blood heat disturbing the *shén*, the *shén* and *hún* separating and the liver-*hún* wandering away.

Sheng di and *Huang lian* were used to cool the blood and clear heat; *Dang gui* was used to nourish the blood; *Duan ci shi* and *Zhu sha* were for settling and calming; and *Gan cao* and *Jian qu* (*Shen qu*) were added to harmonize the stomach.

This patient was cured in a short time due to the precision of the herbal prescription.

---

177 For example, in the *Elementary Questions* Treatises 44 and 60

Menopausal syndrome

Zàng zao-visceral agitation

Forty-one-year-old Mrs. Zhang had had a hysterectomy, including the removal of her left ovary, after a history of endometriosis. After the surgery, she suffered from profuse sweating due to weakness, oedema of the hands and feet, palpitations, insomnia and sadness. Other symptoms included dysphoria, restlessness, intermittent feverishness, chest stuffiness, nausea, poor appetite, distention and pain in the right rib-side, frequent urination and defecation. She had a thin, yellow and greasy tongue coat, and a deep, thin pulse.

The diagnosis was heart and kidney deficiency with liver and stomach disharmony and weakened spleen. The treatment method was to invigorate the heart and kidney, harmonize the liver and stomach and strengthen the spleen. The formula used was Gān mài dà zǎo tāng:

Gan cao (Radix Glycyrrhizae)	6g
Huai xiao mai (Fructus Tritici Aestivi)	15g
Da zao (Fructus Jujubae)	6 pieces

With the addition of other medicinals, such as:

Dang shen (Radix Codonopsis)	12g
Fu ling (Sclerotium Poriae Cocos)	12g
He huan pi (Cortex Albiziae)	12g
Mai dong (Radix Ophiopogonis)	9g
Chen pi (Pericarpium Citri Reticulatae)	6g
Bian dou (Semen Dolichoris)	9g
Zhi xiang fu (prepared Rhizoma Cyperi)	6g
Bai shao (Radix Paeoniae Alba)	9g
Chuan xu duan (Radix Dipsaci)	9g

After three months, all the symptoms were alleviated.

The above case is from Qián Bóxuān Case Studies in Gynaecology (2006), republished from the original People's Medical Publishing House Masters of Chinese Medicine Series (1960s–1980s).

Notes

Qián Bóxuān (b. 1896) was one of modern China's most well-known and respected doctors. In this case, he states that hysteria is mainly caused by depression and anxiety that damage the liver and spleen and create an imbalance between the heart and kidney. The symptoms are sadness, fright, insomnia, repeated yawning, mental restlessness and abnormal behaviors. *Gān mài dà zǎo tāng* from the *Golden Cabinet* is used with the addition of other medicinals to soothe the liver, harmonize the spleen, calm the mind, nourish the kidney and relieve anxiety.

This case pertains to menopausal syndrome. Mrs. Zhang's hysterectomy damaged the *yīn qì*, which led to hyperactivity of *yáng qì*, causing palpitations, feverishness and spontaneous sweating. Sweat is the fluid of the heart. Deficiency of heart *yīn*-blood caused her palpitations, insomnia, mental restlessness and sadness. The spleen controls the four limbs and the weakened spleen led to oedema of the hands and feet. The kidney controls urination and defecation and the kidney deficiency resulted in frequent defecation and urination.

Panic attacks

Bēn tún qì-running piglet qì

A 70-year-old woman had been suffering with paroxysmal abdominal pain and vomiting for one year. She had a painful abdominal mass and before the onset of episodes of pain she felt gas rushing upwards from the abdomen to the epigastric area and she felt as if she was going to die. According to her symptoms this was a case of *bēn tún qì* (奔豚气) disease, and the *Golden Cabinet* describes it as having a sudden onset caused by panic. The patient's illness was a result of her chronic feelings of extreme sorrow after the sudden death of her daughter.

Zhāng Zhòngjǐng's *Guì zhī jiā guì tāng* was prescribed:

Gui zhi (Ramulus Cinnamomi)	15g
Bai shao (Radix Paeoniae Alba)	9g
Zhi gan cao (prepared Radix Glycyrrhizae)	6g
Sheng jiang (Rhizoma Zingiberis Recens)	9g
Da zao (Fructus Jujubae)	4 pieces

After 14 doses, the woman's *bēn tún qì* syndrome was mostly relieved, but she still had abdominal noises and one instance of vomiting. To regulate the stomach and eliminate retained fluids, the same formula was administered with the addition of *Ban xia* (9g) and *Fu ling* (9g).

On her third visit, the woman still had occasional, slight rushing pain in the epigastrium, headache, unsmooth stool and a wiry pulse in the left *guān* position. These symptoms were caused by stomach *qì* counterflow, and the formula was changed to *Lǐ zhōng tāng* (理中汤) with the addition of *Rou guì* and *Wu zhu yu* to warm the stomach and liver. The patient recovered and showed no recurrence after a follow-up inquiry two months later.

The above case is from *Yuè Měizhōng Collected Case Studies* (2007), republished from the original People's Medical Publishing House *Masters of Chinese Medicine Series* (1960s–1980s).

Notes

Yuè Měizhōng (1900–1982), a well-known doctor and professor of Chinese medicine, was for some time responsible for the healthcare of China's senior leaders. In this case, his close study of Zhāng Zhòngjǐng's work led to the application of a *bēn tún qì* strategy given in the *Golden Cabinet*, Chapter 8 (Line 8.3). In the *Treatise on Cold Damage*, the same formula is recommended for *tàiyáng* diseases where excessive sweating has caused dispersal of the heart *yáng* and accelerated the ascent of *yáng* from the lower *jiāo*.

The *Guì zhī* formulas, *Guì zhī tāng*, *Guì zhī jiā guì tāng* and *Guì zhī jiā lóng gǔ mǔ lì tāng*, can be considered in cases where the patient with spontaneous sweating, feverishness, pale face and forceless pulse, experiences a subjective feeling of pulsating, upward movement in the body trunk. Heart or aortic palpitations, or a feeling of movement in the abdomen, all conform to the running piglet *qì* main symptom. This kind of upsurging *qì* counterflow, especially when accompanied by fear, fright or nervousness with restlessness and insomnia, clearly indicates *bēn tún qì* disease.

Yuè Měizhōng uses his deep knowledge of Zhāng Zhòngjǐng's work to explain why the additional *Guì* (Cinnamomi) in this formula is not *Rou guì*. *Guì zhī* is more appropriate for heart and chest *yáng* deficiency and *Rou gui* for a more systemic *yáng* vacuity involving the lifegate fire. In this case, the shock and sorrow of the patient's loss has damaged her chest and heart *yáng*, including the *shén–pò*, and when the *yáng* of the upper *jiāo* is weakened it can no longer control the upward movement of *yáng qì*. In subsequent treatments, Yuè does administer *Rou guì* as part of a *Lǐ zhōng tāng* strategy to strengthen the patient's middle *jiāo yáng* transformations.

Yuè also uses his deployment of *Guì zhī jiā gui tāng* in this case to demonstrate the importance of not only the choice and specificity of medicinals, but also their dosage. A change in dosage of one medicinal can augment the power of the formula, or even change its function. Increasing the dose of *Gui zhi* (Ramulus Cinnamomi) from 9 grams in *Guì zhī tāng* changes the formula from one that treats the *Tai yáng* wind stroke syndrome (with signs and symptoms of sweating, fever and aversion to wind more than cold), to one that can cure *bēn tún qì* disease due to heart *yáng* vacuity, *Guì zhī jiā guì tāng*.

Turbid phlegm fire leading to insanity

Turbid phlegm fire enters the liver, *hún* wandering insanity

Mr. Wu worked in Hubei province and had a strange problem: he talked to and reviled non-living things such as food, clothes and utensils. He sought treatment far and wide, but his problem was regarded as an evil attack that could not be cured. He eventually asked for permission to return to his home town for treatment.

When he came to see me,[178] I felt that his left *guān* pulse was thready, wiry and slippery, which indicated phlegm fire entering the liver, causing the liver to fail in its storing of the *hún* and the *hún* wandering away. This problem is not an evil attack. I used some herbs to clear fire, dissolve phlegm and to suppress the excess *yáng* and adverse *qì*.

The prescription contained:

Ling yáng jiao (Cornu Saigae Tataricae)^	3g
Shi jue ming (Concha Haliotidis)	12g
Dan pi (Cortex Moutan)	6g
Chuan bei mu (Bulbus Fritillariae Cirrhosae)	9g

---

178 费伯雄 Fèi Bóxióng (1810–1877), the most famous exponent of the Mèng hé school (Scheid 2007)

Shi hu (Herba Dendrobii)^	9g
Tian hua fen (Radix Trichosanthis)	9g
Mai dong (Radix Ophiopogonis)	9g
Long chi (Dens Draconis)	9g
Ju hong (Pericarpium Citri Reticulatae)	3g
Zhu li (Succus Bambusae)	6g

(^ CITES Endangered species)

After taking six bags of this prescription, the problem was cured.

The liver stores the *hún*, but when phlegm fire disturbs the liver it causes the liver *yáng* to rise. The *hún* is unsettled and wanders away, and it becomes attached to things outside one's person. Medicinals that clear fire and dissolve phlegm subdue excess liver *yáng* so that the *shén* and *hún* may be stored properly. There is no similar case recorded in any of the ancient classics; however, pulse diagnosis and pattern identification enable the borrowing of treatment ideas for extensive applications.

The above is 'The Case of Mr. Qi,' from the 'Strange Diseases' section in the *Mèng hé Medical Cases* (*c.* 1850–1875), Yu Tinghong Publishing House (first edition: Qing Dynasty); Shanghai Science and Technology Press (second edition: April 2010).[179]

Notes from Zǔ Yí[180]

The prescription borrows ideas from one of Dr. Xu's cases, and uses a modified version of the *Zhēn zhū mǔ wán* formula together with modified *Xún lóng tāng* to treat wandering *hún*. The case was recorded in the *Supplementary Notions of Medical Experience*[181] (1863) by Fèi Bóxióng, and indicates that *Zhēn zhū mǔ wán* is a miracle formula to treat liver *hún* disorders.

---

179 《孟河费式医案 · 孟河费绳甫先生医案 · 奇病》 *Mèng hé fèi shì yī àn, 'Mèng hé fèi shéng fǔ xiān shēng yī àn,' 'Qí bìng'* (费伯雄(清代) 余听鸿出版社 (初版: 上海科学技术出版社再版; 2010 年 04月)
180 祖怡 Zǔ Yí, a commentator on the Mèng hé cases
181 《医醇賸义》 *Yī chún shèng yì*

Notes

The left *guān* pulse represents liver and the thready, wiry and slippery qualities indicate phlegm fluid retention. The pulse on the left side is the main point identifying the pattern. It reflects the patho-mechanism whereby phlegm fire disrupts the liver causing uncontrolled liver *yáng* to rise up. This causes the *shén* and the *hún* to wander away and become attached to other things. Therefore, the patient talks to these other things.

The heart stores the *shén*, and the liver stores the *hún*; the heart opens to the tongue and the liver to the eyes; talking is the activity of the heart and seeing is the activity of the liver.

In the *Divine Pivot*, Treatise 8 says that the *hún* comes and goes with the *shén*, so normally the *shén* and *hún* accompany one another. In disorder, the *shén* and *hún* separate and the *hún* wanders like a ghost. The person presents as mentally deranged and delirious, talking wildly.

Ling yáng jiao, *Mu dan pi*, *Chuan bei mu*, *Ju hong* and *Zhu li* are used to clear fire and dissolve phlegm.

Shi hu, *Tian hua fen*, *Mai men dong*, *Long chi* and *Shi jue ming* nourish the *yīn* and subdue excess *yáng*.

The prescription was able to help retrieve and settle the *shén* and *hún*, so then the phantasma and delirium stopped and the strange problem was cured.

Psychosis

Mania for seven years after thwarted ambition

Mr. Bao, 32 years old, had severe psychosis for seven years after he failed to succeed in the imperial examinations. He had undergone treatment with many doctors, including expert physicians in the Beijing City and Confucian Hospitals. He also consulted dozens of doctors from his home town Huizhou, as well as Hangzhou, Suzhou and Hubei Hospitals. Most of the treatments tried supplementation, a few used reducing methods. Some worked for a short time and he felt well and normal; however, positive effects were always short-lived.

When I (Wú Jūtōng)[182] first saw him, his face was dirty, his hair disheveled and he was in rags. His genitals, which appeared totally red, were exposed. Wherever he went, there was chaos and mess. His

---

182 吴鞠通 Wú Jūtōng (1757–1841)

family had to keep him in an empty room, with his hands and feet chained to a large grindstone because he had smashed and destroyed the doors and windows and removed all their nails. He was thin and weak, and in a state of confusion. If his wife refused to see him daily as he demanded, Bao would fly into a rage. He would yell himself hoarse and wail so unbearably that the family would have to ask maids and concubines to serve him so that he would calm down. But he would soon resume his uproar and this continued day after day.

I felt his pulse and found that all six positions were taut, long and powerful. The pulse indicated that Mr. Bao had a repletion rather than a depletion illness and I gave him the bitterest herbs in order to clear heat from the heart and small intestine. In some cases, when the *zàng* have problems, we treat their interiorly–exteriorly related *fǔ*. According to this theory, I cleared the man's heart heat by purging the stool and urine to clear heat via his intestines.

Long dan cao (Radix Gentianae)   9g

Huang lian (Rhizoma Coptis)   9g

Tian men dong (Radix Asparagi)   9g

Mai men dong (Radix Ophiopogonis)   9g

Sheng di huang (Radix Rehmannia)   9g

Mu dan pi (Cortex Moutan)   9g

Drain after boiling to obtain three cups of decoction, for three doses.

After only two days there was a big change—his crying and raving lessened and he began to behave more quietly, and by the third day the effect of the formula was obvious. However, I thought that because of the long course of the disease, he was too weak to bear the harsh properties of the formula. It is said that too much hardness will result in a break, so I reduced the bitter herbs and added some with sweet and rich properties to nourish *yīn*-fluids. On the fifth day the patient's family sent someone, saying that after taking two doses of the new formula yesterday, he suddenly became much worse. He cried and raved much more again and was unable to calm down for even one minute. His family thought that maybe this kind of disease could not be cured and he was certain to die, and so they asked me not to treat him anymore.

I didn't believe this was the case. The first formula was harsh but had been very effective, and when the gentler *yīn*-nourishing formula was given his condition deteriorated again. It seemed I had initially understood the nature of his symptoms after all. I checked his pulse again, which was still taut, long and rapid, so I increased the content of the bitter herbs.

Long dan cao (Radix Gentianae)	18g
Lu hui (Aloe)^	18g
Huang lian (Coptis Rhizoma)	15g
Tian men dong (Radix Asparagi)	15g
Mai men dong (Radix Ophiopogonis)	15g
Shi hu (Herba Dendrobii)^	6g
Wu mei (Fructus Mume)	15g

Drain after boiling to obtain three cups of decoction, for three doses.

(^ CITES Endangered species)

He took the formula for six days and his condition gradually improved. By day 11 he was clear-headed and could communicate with people, and I was able to tell him why he had become ill. With a narrow view and wrong understanding of beauty and the limits of life, he had absolutely no perspective on the complexity and importance of the supreme realm. He had limited himself to his own desires and when he failed, he flew into a rage. It was so fortunate to live in the world; how could he be angry with his circumstances? What's more, one of the most important things in life is to honor and take care of our parents.

Hearing my criticism, he bent his head and said nothing. As the days passed, I reduced the bitter herbs of the formula and added some that would nourish the *yīn*. After half a month, the chains were removed, he dressed himself carefully and kneeled to express his gratitude to me. By this time, he was as normal as everyone else. Thereafter by taking Special Harmonizing and Vitalizing Paste he became stronger and stronger, and unexpectedly succeeded in the imperial examination in the following year.

The above is taken from the 'Mania' section in *Wú Jūtōng's Medical Records*,[183] Qing Dynasty (1644–1911).

Notes

Wú Jūtōng was an admirer of Yè Tiānshì[184] (1667–1746) and his work on Warm Diseases (温病 *wēn bìng*), although the Special Harmonizing and Vitalizing Paste[185] was of Wú Jūtōng's own invention. The paste contains dozens of ingredients and Wú often used it at the end of his Warm Disease treatments to replenish and balance the *yīn* and *yáng*.

Wú Jūtōng's case records note that social and emotional frustrations could cause serious madness, and that Mr. Bao 'had first become ill because his achievements did not follow his ambitions.' The case illustrates the links between mental–emotional factors and mental illness, and the importance given to both medication and advice in the treatment of mental–emotional disorders by Chinese physicians in the Qing.

Bao's disappointments had turned into an internal repletion fire that Wú Jūtōng was able to clear using bitter and cold purgative medicinals. After repeated doses, Bao had recovered sufficiently for Wú to reproach him and to urge him to remember the importance of filial behavior.

Bao had failed his family by reacting angrily to his disappointment, and the re-assertion of proper social and family roles was part of Wú Jūtōng's efficacious treatment in this case. Wú's emphasis on the value of traditional roles and responsibilities afforded Bao a social position that did not depend on examination success and reaffirmed the culturally powerful notion of filial piety as more important than individual achievements.

Depressive psychosis

Overly suspicious and anxious, leading to phlegm constraint madness

Mr. Wang once treated a lady who suspected that her husband was in love with another woman, as a consequence of which, she went crazy. She talked incessantly day and night, turned around and around at

---

183 《吴鞠通医案 · 癫狂》 *Wú Jūtōng yī àn, Diān kuáng*
184 叶天士 Yè Tiānshì
185 专翕大生膏 *Zhuān xī dà shēng gāo*

home, and no one could catch her. Mr. Wang prescribed 80 'Vaporize Phlegm Pills.'[186] After taking them, she could sleep without any talking, and then she took another 80 pills. Following each of the two rounds of pills, she passed a large bowel movement that eliminated evil stuff. The lady blushed with shame; however, she was able to return to her normal life.

To prevent a recurrence, Mr. Wang asked someone to chat with another person who stood right next to the lady. When she overheard them saying that the woman who her husband loved had just died suddenly from summer heat, the lady felt excited and asked how the man knew about it. He replied that he personally saw the woman's husband preparing for her funeral. Mr. Wang's patient then felt happy and was cured.

At the same time, Mr. Wang spoke with his patient's family to check if she was having a normal period. Her aunty said that the lady's period had stopped months ago because she wasn't eating and had lost weight. Mr. Wang asked the family to come by and pick up some herbs to nourish the lady's blood and restore her period. Her family followed the instructions and for half a month she took 'Harmonious Marriage Nourish Blood Decoction'[187] for amenorrhea, followed by a modified 'Four Substances Decoction'[188] to nourish the blood. Finally, she was fine and never had the same problem again.

It is noted that whoever starts the trouble should end it. There once was a patient who became sick due to poverty. The doctor asked someone to deliver a lot of money and riches to this patient, which cured him. However, this was a matter of expediency. Deception can only be a temporary measure because once patients realize the ploy, they become sick again.

Patients must be helped with appropriate consultation. The doctor should enlighten their patients so that after their condition is clarified and they realize their problems, they will not become sick again. There was another patient who experienced hallucinations and saw things like lions. Mr. Yi Chuan taught this patient to try and catch what he saw with his hands. When the patient found he could touch nothing at all, he was gradually cured.

---

186 滚痰丸 *Gǔn tán wán* ('Vaporize Phlegm Pills,' also known as *Méng shí gǔn tán wán* or 'Lapis and Scute Vaporize Phlegm Pills')
187 婚合门中滋血汤 *Hūn hé mén zhōng zī xuè tāng*
188 四物汤 *Sì wù tāng*

This is a holy and sincere thought for people to learn, but realization is easily confused and implementation hard to achieve. Only if every doctor can treat the root of the problem and focus on the cause, can Xuān Yuán and Qí Bó's thoughts be truly passed down.

The above case is from *Ancient and Modern Medical Cases*, 'Madness'[189] (1778).

Notes

Over-suspicion and anxiety upset the *shén*, block *qì* movement and generate phlegm accumulation. When the heart fails to store the *shén*, the patient may talk constantly and not sleep at all.

Gǔn tán wán was used to clear phlegm fire and open the apertures. This restores the *shén*, which in turn normalizes the patient's sleeping and communication. The bowel movements that eliminated the pathogenic factors also helped to recover the lady's *shén*. Although she felt ashamed, purgation actually cleared and removed repletion evils so that no more reducing treatments were needed. Subsequently, and in consideration of this lady's actual problem, a form of psychological therapy was used.

The lady's real problem was psychological, and when she became happy it indicated her suspicion and anxiety had gone and she was cured. In the end, and to help complete the treatment and prevent recurrence, only some caring thoughts and suggestions were needed.

Postpartum depressive psychosis

Juéyīn static blood and heat, turbid phlegm obstructs the stomach

Sometimes after giving birth there can be mental disorder that begins with madness, delirium and laughing, and the patient's condition then changes so that they look like dead wood. The problem is due to static blood and heat entering the *juéyīn*, together with turbid phlegm obstructing the stomach. The illness can persist and gradually consolidate over several years. It can become so firmly entrenched it cannot be helped by light interventions.

The recommended prescription is:

---

189 《古今医案按 · 癫狂》 *Gǔ jīn yī àn àn, Diān kuáng*

4.5 grams of *Méng shí gǔn tán wán* (Lapis and Scute Vaporize Phlegm Pills)[190] taken on an empty stomach just before sleep.

and a decoction of four herbs:

Dan shen (Radix Salviae Miltiorrhizae)

Tao ren (Semen Persicae)

Su mu (Lignum Sappan)

Jiang xiang (Lignum Dalbergiae Odiferae)^

Drained after boiling to obtain two doses, and taken just before sleep.

(^ CITES Endangered species)

The above is from the *Liǔ Bǎoyi Medical Records*, 'Shén zhì'[191] (1965).

Notes

After giving birth, the mother's *yīn*-blood is suddenly depleted and this can lead to a state of hyperactive *yáng* madness. Giving birth can also cause static blood that can combine with phlegm to block the heart-*shén* aperture. The illness manifests with mental derangement and a state of withdrawal as if the patient is like dead wood. This is similar nowadays to postpartum psychosis and depression.

Méng shí gǔn tán wán dissolves phlegm and opens the heart aperture. *Dan shen*, *Tao ren*, *Su mu* and *Jiang xiang* are aromatic, promote blood circulation and remove stasis. They gradually break up the consolidated stagnation to open the heart-*shén* aperture. When the aperture is open, the clear *shén* is retrieved and the problem is cured.

---

190 Same as *Gǔn tán wán* in the previous case
191 《柳宝诒医案 · 神志》 *Liǔ Bǎoyí yī àn, Shénzhì* ((清)柳宝诒著 人民卫生出版社 出版时间: 1965) ((*Qīng*) *Liǔ Bǎoyí zhù Rénmín Wèishēng Chūbǎn shè chūbǎn shíjiān*: 1965)

Appendix 1:
Acupuncture Points

Acupuncture points are known to adjust the *qì*, and acupuncture therapy will therefore be as useful for psychological illnesses as it is for so many other conditions. Properly trained acupuncture practitioners perform Chinese medicine diagnoses as described in the chapters above. The selection of points for treatment then relies on a deep understanding of channel theory, point dynamics and palpatory diagnostics.

The conditions listed below roughly follow the categories discussed in Part 2. The acupuncture points are listed using the World Health Organization's standard abbreviations for the 14 main channels. Practitioners will recognize the points in this section as commonly recommended and experientially useful for mental and emotion-related disorders. The points listed are not prescriptions and are meant only as a reminder of possible selections when designing a treatment prescription according to Chinese medicine and channel diagnosis. The points here are by no means an exhaustive list of the practitioner's options for their acupuncture prescriptions.

That said, we recommend the front *mu*-alarm points and back *shu*-transport points for their direct connections with the interior, and with specific *zàng fǔ* systems and their senses. They can be selected for any *zàng shén* disharmony and combined with appropriate *shu*-transport points on the main channels. For example, for liver-*hún* disorders, LR14 or BL18 may be combined with LR2, LR3 or LR8 to address liver fire repletion, *qì* constraint or liver *yīn* depletion patterns, and so on.

According to channel theory, the bladder channel and governing vessel have connections with the kidney-lifegate and the brain, and they both carry the kidney-lifegate's *yáng qì* and source *qì* influences to the *zàng fǔ* visceral systems. This makes both channels very useful for *shén zhì* disease treatments. GV24 calms the *shén*, GV4 invigorates lifegate fire and BL66 quietens the mind, for example; and one of the governing vessel's classic dysfunctions is a rushing sensation from the lower abdomen up to the chest and heart, similar to the *bēn tún qì* disorder.

The back *shu*-transport points can be combined with their outer bladder channel points (such as BL42 'Door of the *pò*,' and BL44 'Hall of the *shén*'), and/or with one another to benefit *zàng shén* activities. For example, BL23 with BL52 strengthens the lower back and the kidney-*zhì*; and BL15 with BL23 harmonizes the heart-*shén* and kidney-*zhì*.

Suggestions for auricular acupuncture are shown next to the 𝔖 symbol, and suggestions for moxa treatments are shown next to the △ symbol. Moxibustion treatments are recommended for *qì* or *yáng qì* depletion or phlegm dampness or cold illness patterns. Additional information on points and prescriptions, the extra (non-channel) points and auricular points, needling techniques and moxibustion protocols are available in many English translations and textbooks, some of which are noted below in 'References and Further Reading.'

Agitation: *An mian* (extra point), CV17, LU4, ST23, ST41, SP1, SP2, KD1, KD4, PC4, PC7, GB8, GB12

Anger: GV8, BL18, BL47, LR14, CV14, PC8, LR2

Anxiety: *Yin tang* (extra point), GV11, GV20, GV24, CV14, BL15, BL44, GB43; HT7 with BL60
𝔖 Shenmen, Subcortex, Sympathetic, Brain, Endocrine, Heart, Spleen, Liver, Kidney

Dementia: *Yin tang, Si shén cong* (extra points), CV4, CV6, CV17, GV4, GV14, GV16, the 'sea of marrow' (GV16 with GV20), BL15, BL18, BL23, HT7, PC6, PC7, KD4, ST36, ST40
△ LI4, LI5, LI11, LU10, HT3, HT7, BL13, LR2, BL64

Depletion taxation: CV4, CV6, GV4, BL23, BL43, GB19; the 'sea of nourishment' (ST36 with ST30)
△ *Si hua xue* (BL17 with BL19); ST36, BL42, BL43, CV4, CV6

Depression: CV14, GV15, GV24, GV26, BL15, BL17, BL18, HT5, HT7, PC6, LR3, LR5, ST40; GB13 with GB9 and GB36; SJ6 with LR2
△ CV4, CV6, GV20, BL23, LR3, ST36
𝔇 Shenmen, Subcortex, Brain, Heart, Spleen, Liver, Kidney

Dreams (excessive dreaming, nightmares): BL14, BL15, BL18, KD3, KD6, TE16, SP5, GB11; (with depression) *Si shén cong* with GV8 and BL18; (and easily startled) HT7 with BL15 and ST44

Fearful: *Yin tang* (extra point), GV16, HT4, GB9; GB34 with KD2; GB34 with HT7 and PC6; (susceptible to fright) BL18 with BL19 and BL66
△ KD2, LR2, GB43, PC6 and SP9

Forgetful (poor memory): *Si shen cong* (extra points), CV14, GV11, BL15, BL20, BL23, BL43, HT3, HT7, PC6, GB20, KD3, KD7
△ GV20, CV12, BL15, HT3, HT7, LU7, ST36

Insomnia: *An mian, Yin tang, Si shen cong* (extra points), GV19, GV20, GV24, BL15, BL19, BL62, KD6, SP6, HT7, PC6, GB12, GB20, GB23; GV11 with HT7 and SP6; BL62 with HT7 or KD3
𝔇 Shenmen, Subcortex, Spleen, Liver, Kidney

Lily disease: CV14, BL13, BL15, BL23, HT6, LU6, LU9, KD3, KD6, SP6; (hunger but no desire to eat) Needle and △ LR13 and LR14

Mania: *Si shén cong, Shi xuan* (extra points), CV13, CV14, CV15, GV8, GV12, GV16, GV20, GV26, HT7, PC6, PC7, GB12, SI3, KD1, ST40, BL66, TE2; SI3 with BL62; BL64 with SP6 and ST40; (clear heart fire, calm the *shén*) ST23 or ST24 with GV20
𝔇 Sympathetic, Shenmen, Subcortex, Brain, Heart, Spleen, Liver, Kidney, Endocrine, Brain

Manic depression: *Si shén cong* (extra points), CV14, GV15, BL15, BL62, BL65, ST40, PC8, GB19, GB21, GB24; GV13 and GV26 with BL13 and BL17; (for mania and insanity-withdrawal) KD10, BL62 and BL64

Menopausal syndrome: CV4, CV6, GV4, GV14, GV20, BL18, BL20, BL23, HT7, SP6, ST36; (with night sweats) KD3 with HT6; (with hypertension) LI11 with LR3
𝔇 Endocrine, Subcortex, Ovary, Shenmen, Heart, Kidney, Occiput, Uterus

Palpitations (due to fright): BL15, HT7, PC6, GB19, CV7; PC7 with ST36
🔊 Heart, Subcortex, Sympathetic

Plum pit *qì* (globus hystericus): CV12, CV14, CV17, ST40, HT5, HT7, HT8, KD6, PC5, LR3, LR5, LI4, LI18, LU10; LR3 with CV17 and CV22; or, KD6 with CV17 and CV22; (with difficulty swallowing) ST9

Postpartum exhaustion: (Needle and △) *Bai lao* (extra point) with CV3, CV6, SP6, BL12 and BL23

Psychosis (schizophrenia, madness): GV8, GV16, GV18, BL5, BL60, ST40, KD9, LR2, GB9; GB13 with GV12; GV23 with BL45 and TE16
△ LU11, CV4, CV12, CV14

Running piglet *qì* disease: CV3, CV4, CV5, CV7, CV17, CV18, GV5, PC6; SI3 with GV4
△ CV3, CV6, LR14

Sadness: GV11, GV13, GV20, LU3, LU9, ST36, HT7, PC6; (with sighing) GB23 with GB24 and SP5

Sea of marrow (the brain, the mansion of *jīng*-essence, depleted): GV4, GV20, BL23, BL60, KD3, HT7; the 'sea of marrow' (GV16 with GV20)

Thinking (excessive): SP5, LR13, BL20, Bl49

Worry (excessive): CV12, BL13, BL20, BL49

Vexation (heart/mind restless and irritable due to heat): HT3, HT6, HT7, PC3, PC6, PC7

Visceral agitation: *Si shén cong* (extra points), GV8, BL14, HT4, HT5, HT7, SI7, PC8, SP6, ST40; GV26 with PC6; GB9 with SP15; KD6 with PC6 and GV26; PC6 with GV20 and GV26; (with aphasia) HT5, or ST9 with CV23
🔊 Heart, Kidney, Brain stem, Shenmen, Occiput, Subcortex, Sympathetic

Appendix 2: Glossary
of Chinese Terms

Characters	Pinyin	English
白合病	*bái hé bìng*	Lily bulb disease or hundred union disease
本神	*běn shén*	The root *shén*, the root of the postnatal *shén*, the source of sentient life and human mentality Also known as the source *shén* (原神 *yuán shén*)
奔豚气病	*bēn tún qì bìng*	Running piglet *qì* disease, the main illness category discussed in Chapter 8 of the *Golden Cabinet* 'Running piglet' describes the feeling of *qì* ascending from the lower *jiāo* to the chest and throat Associated with panic attacks, fear, fright and anger
蔽	*bì*	Cover, conceal, obsession, blindness
不明	*bù míng*	Without brightness, unenlightened, dark and irrational, dull and confused
陈言	Chén Yán	1131–1139, author of *Discussion of Illnesses, Patterns, and Formulas Related to the Unification of the Three Aetiologies* (1173)
道	*dào*	Law, cosmic law, law of nature, way of nature Way, pathway, road Way of living (stillness, softness, humility) The state of nothingness, before space and time
道德经	*Dào dé jīng*	*Classic of the Law/The Way and its Power*, c. 460 BCE, attributed to Lǎo Zǐ
道象器	*dào xiàng qì*	Law, phenomenon and entity Three levels of reality discussed in the *Book of Changes*' commentaries

cont.

Characters	Pinyin	English
得神者昌，失神者亡	*Dé shén zhě chāng, shī shén zhě wáng*	'Life flourishes with *shén*; Life perishes without *shén*' (from the *Inner Canon, Elementary Questions* Treatise 13)
癫狂	*diān kuáng*	Severe mental disorder, insanity-withdrawal, depressive psychosis, schizophrenia, mania
动气	*dòng qì*	Dynamic *qì*, moving *qì* The dynamic *qì* is located beneath the level of the navel and between the kidneys The name given by the *Classic of Difficult Issues*, Issue 8, it is the source of the channels and *zàng fǔ*
分	*fēn*	Share, allotment
封藏	*fēng cáng*	Seal and store (kidney *zàng* function)
傅青主	Fù Qīngzhǔ	1607–1684, author of *Fù Qīngzhǔ's Gynaecology* (first published in 1826)
官	*guān*	Office, administrative post the *Inner Canon*'s twelve palace officials (*Elementary Questions*, Treatise 8) The five senses, as administrative officials and their offices, i.e. the eyes, ears, tongue (taste and speech), nose and skin
光	*guāng*	Light, luminescence
归根	*guīgēn*	Root-tendency
归根心理学	*guīgēn xīnlǐ xué*	Root-tendency psychology, a recent branch of TCM psychology
后天	*hòu tiān*	Postnatal, post-heavenly, acquired, after birth
黄帝内经	*Huáng dì nèi jīng*	*Yellow Emperor's Inner Canon* (*c.* 100 BCE) There are two parts to the *Inner Canon*: the *Elementary Questions* and the *Divine Pivot*, each with 81 treatises
黄帝阴符经 (黄帝陰符經)	*Huáng dì yīn fú jīng*	*The Yellow Emperor's Hidden Talisman Canon* (*c.* 8th century CE), a Daoist text associated with inner cultivation
魂	*hún*	Soul, sometimes *yáng* soul, ethereal soul or sentient soul (According to the *Book of Changes*, 'The *shén* cannot be measured by *yīn* and *yáng*') Lodges in the liver *zàng* Participates in the function of the eyes (vision, eyesight) and the sinews (movement, balance)

Characters	Pinyin	English
混元气	*hùn yuán qì*	*Qì* monism From nothingness (the *dào*) comes 'the one,' the primary or primordial *qì*, the basis of all phenomena in the universe Myriad things all arise from this one *qì*
金匮要略	*Jīn guì yào lüè*	*Essential Prescriptions of the Golden Cabinet*, by Zhāng Zhòngjǐng, originally *c.* 220 CE
金匮要略·五脏风寒积聚病	*Jīn guì yào lüè, Wǔ zàng fēng hán jī jù bìng*	*Essential Prescriptions of the Golden Cabinet*, 'Wind and Cold in the Five *Zàng* and Accumulations and Gatherings' (Chapter 11)
积神于心，以知往今	*Jī shén yú xīn, yǐ zhī wǎng jīn*	'*Shén* accumulates in the heart, it knows the past and the present' (from the *Divine Pivot*, Treatise 49)
近朱者赤，近墨者黑	*Jìn zhū zhě chì, jìn mò zhě hēi*	'Close to cinnabar you are red [loyal and sincere], close to ink you are black [dark]' (Chinese saying)
精	*jīng*	Essence, one of Chinese medicine's *qì*-substances, a refined concentrate of *qì* stored in the kidneys The term usually includes prenatal (inherited) and postnatal (acquired) *jīng*-essence *Jīng*-essence is responsible for growth, development and reproduction
精气神	*jīng qì shén*	Essence *qì shén* The 'three treasures' (*sān bǎo* 三宝)
精神	*jīng shén*	Essence and *shén*
厥气	*jué qì*	Reversing *qì*, disturbed or disorderly *qì* movement The *qì* moves contrary to its regular course
君主	*jūn zhǔ*	Sovereign ruler, eminent ruler, monarch
刻骨铭心	*Kè gǔ míng xīn*	'Engraved in the bones and imprinted on the heart' (Chinese saying) A memory or experience that deeply influences the heart-*shén*; it leaves its mark, or is deposited in, the deeper aspects of the *shén*
老子	Lǎo Zǐ	Dates unknown, sixth century BCE, thought to have written the *Dào dé jīng*
类经	*Lèi jīng*	*Classified Canon* (1624), by Zhāng Jièbīn
理	*lǐ*	Principle, texture Rational, logical and reasonable

cont.

Characters	Pinyin	English
理性	*lǐ xìng*	Rational, rationality Problems and issues are dealt with in a balanced way using the principles of *yīn–yáng*
理智	*lǐ zhì*	*Lǐ* is logical, rational and reasonable, *zhì* is wisdom and moral intelligence
礼 (禮)	*lǐ*	Propriety, courtesy
李时珍	Lǐ Shízhēn	1518–1593, author of the *Compendium of Materia Medica* 本草纲目 *běn cǎo gāng mù*
灵	*líng*	Divine, miraculous, luminous, holy
灵枢	*Líng shū*	The *Divine Pivot*, the second part of the *Inner Canon*, *c.* 100 BCE
灵枢·本神	*Líng shū, Běn shén*	*Divine Pivot*, 'The Root [of the] *Shen*' (Treatise 8)
灵枢·淫邪发梦	*Líng shū, Yín xié fā mèng*	*Divine Pivot*, 'Excess Evils Release Dreams' (Treatise 43)
灵枢·五色	*Líng shū, Wǔ sè*	*Divine Pivot*, 'Five Colours [Complexions]' (Treatise 49)
灵枢·天年	*Líng shū, Tiān nián*	*Divine Pivot*, 'Years Given by Heaven' (Treatise 54)
灵枢·阴阳二十五人	*Líng shū, Yīn yáng èr shí wǔ rén*	*Divine Pivot*, 'Yīn Yáng and the Twenty-five Human Types' (Treatise 64)
灵枢·通天	*Líng shū, Tōng tiān*	*Divine Pivot*, 'Connecting Heaven' (Treatise 72)
吕洞宾	Lǚ Dòngbīn	Tang dynasty Daoist adept (798–?)
论语	*Lún yǔ*	*Analects of Confucius* (*c.* 475–221 BCE)
毛泽东	Máo Zédōng	1893–1976, founding leader of the People's Republic of China (1949–)
梅核气	*méi hé qì*	Plum pit *qì* An emotion-related illness whose characteristic feature is the sensation of something lodged in the throat *Globus hystericus*

Characters	Pinyin	English
蒙	*méng*	Covered, blindfolded, veiled, dark, dim, irrational 蒙昧 *Méng mèi*—veiled and dark, uncultured and ignorant; an expression that means there is little intelligence (*ming*-brightness) when one is born *Méng mèi* is the opposite of *míng xī* (see below)
梦游	*mèng yóu*	Excess dreaming (that disturbs normal sleep), due to frenetic wandering of the *hún* at night Sleepwalking, night walking, nightmares, a form of *shén–hún* disharmony causing *hún–pò* wandering 梦呓 *Mèng yì*—talking while asleep, can be a sign of psychological pressure, but is a less serious disturbance affecting only the heart-*shén* and tongue
孟子	Mèng Zǐ	Mencius, *c.* 372–289 BCE, Confucian philosopher
迷	*mí*	Confused, lost, fascinated, fixated, obsessed
命	*mìng*	Life, destiny, fate
命门	*mìng mén*	The lifegate The root and source of life within the kidneys after birth
明	*míng*	Clear, bright, radiant, brilliant On the left side of the character is the sun and on the right side is the moon—together they radiate light night and day so we never lose our way
明君	*míng jūn*	Exceptional qualities A wise governor
明晰	*míng xī*	*Míng* means bright, and *xī* is an accomplished ability for analysis, discernment and judgment *Míng xī*—having good judgment, rational intelligence, [the person is] never in a dark state *Míng xī* is the opposite of *méng mèi*
明心	*míng xīn*	Heart brightness and enlightenment
明心见性	*ming xīn jiàn xìng*	Heart (spirit/mind) brightness reveals our inner nature and natural qualities
难经	*Nán jīng*	*Canon of Difficult Issues* (first century CE), author/s unknown
内伤	*nèi shāng*	Inner harm Illness due to hunger, exhaustion and/or mental–emotional factors

cont.

Characters	Pinyin	English
魄	*pò*	Soul, sometimes *yīn* soul or corporeal soul (According to the *Book of Changes*, 'The *shén* cannot be measured by *yīn* and *yáng*') Lodges in the lung *zàng* Participates in the sensory functions of the nose and skin (olfactory and tactile sensations)
气	*qì*	In medicine, '*qì*' refers to physiological activities, transformations, movements, substances and process events Translations include: influences; function, power, vitalities, energies; air, breath, finest matter; physiological structure, configurational energy
气化	*qì huà*	*Qì* transformations Higher-level physiology and cell metabolism governed by the kidney-lifegate
气机	*qì jī*	*Qì* mechanism or *qì* dynamic *Qì* movement, the correct ascending, descending, sinking and floating movement of *qì*
气立	*qì lì*	*Qì* set-up, or *qì* establishment The climatic conditions, rhythms and cycles of the natural environment The cycles of generation, growth, transformation, harvest and storage that affect all biology, including the physiological movements and transformations of human life Thus, in Chinese medicine we say that human life corresponds to heaven
潜意识	*qián yì shí*	The unconscious mind
窍	*qiào*	Aperture, orifice, opening 开窍 *kāi qiào* means 'opens at' (e.g. the liver opens at the eyes)
情	*qíng*	Emotion, disposition, affect, sentiment, feeling
情志	*qíng zhì*	Emotion, emotional state, disposition
情志病	*qíng zhì bìng*	Emotion-related illness
仁	*rén*	Benevolence, humanity, kindness
人神	*rén shén*	Human life, human being/s

Characters	Pinyin	English
人知其神之神，而不知不神之所以神	*Rén zhī qí shén zhī shén, ér bù zhī bù shén zhī suǒ yǐ shén*	'People know the *shén* of *shén*, but they do not know the no *shén* of the *shén*' (from the *Hidden Talisman Canon*)
三宝	*sān bǎo*	The three treasures The essence, *qì* and spirit/mind (精气神 *jīng qì shén*)
三焦	*sān jiāo*	Triple burner, triple energizer, three heater The upper, middle and lower burning spaces (上焦, 中焦, 下焦 *shàng jiāo, zhōng jiāo, xià jiāo*) *Sān jiāo* arises from the lifegate and distributes the source *qì* (原气 *yuán qì*) throughout the body via its network of spaces and textures (腠理 *còu lǐ*) (see Garvey 2015)
伤寒论	*Shāng hán lùn*	*Treatise on Cold Damage*, by Zhāng Zhòngjǐng, originally *c.* 220 CE
伤寒杂病论	*Shāng hán zá bìng lùn*	*Treatise on Cold Damage and Miscellaneous Diseases* by Zhāng Zhòngjǐng, *c.* 220 CE Nowadays in the form of two books: *Treatise on Cold Damage* and *Essential Prescriptions of the Golden Cabinet*
神	*shén*	Spirit, mind Human mentality and conscious awareness, sentient life
神, 不神	*shén, bù shén*	'Spirit/mind,' and 'no spirit/mind' (terms used in the *Hidden Talisman Canon*) Synonymous with the acquired *shén* and initiating *shén* (terms used in the *Golden Flower*) Both sets of terms are similar to modern psychology's conscious and unconscious mind
神道	*shén dào*	The way of the *shén*, the pathways of the *shén* coming and going Same as 使道 *shǐ dào*—the *Elementary Questions* Treatise 8 uses 使道 for the *shén qì* pathways
神机	*shén jī*	*Shén* dynamic, or *shén* mechanism The innumerable mechanisms of the living body, the generative processes producing life The 'unfathomable transformations of *yīn* and *yáng*'
神明	*shén míng*	*Shén*-spirit/mind brightness and clarity Radiance and brilliance Intelligence and rationality

cont.

Characters	Pinyin	English
神窍	shén qiào	The shén (spirit/mind) aperture, which receives and coordinates sensory information from all the senses Similar to the 心窍 xīn qiào, the aperture of the heart-shén The shén aperture includes all the apertures, the eyes, nose, mouth, ears, tongue, the two yīn apertures in the lower jiāo and the sweat pores of the skin The heart-shén governs all the apertures
神色	shén sè	The observed (diagnostic) manifestations of the shén A person's facial expression and demeanor, their complexion
神遊	shén yóu	Shén wandering
神志	shén zhì	Mind Abbreviated from the five zàng shén, the heart-shén, liver-hún, lung-pò, spleen-yì and kidney-zhì
神志病	shén zhì bìng	Mental illness, mental–emotional disorder, psychological disease
神之神	shén zhī shén	The shén of shén (a term from the Hidden Talisman Canon) Postnatal conscious awareness
身	shēn	Body, self, person, whole person
身体	shén tǐ	Body–person, physical form
身心疾病	shén xīn jí bìng	Body–mind (somato-psychic) disease Physical illness that develops or worsens due to psychological stresses or emotional disturbances
生气	shēng qì	Generative qì, life qì, life force, vitality
识神	shí shén	The acquired shén, postnatal conscious awareness 'Ordinary consciousness'—a term from the Secret of the Golden Flower 神识 Shén shí—recognition and understanding relies on: 鼻识 bí shí—olfactory perception 耳识 ěr shí—auditory perception 舌识 shé shí—taste perception 身识 shēn shí—tactile perception 眼识 yǎn shí—visual perception The orderly coordinated functions of these five are the 'conscious awareness' (意识 yì shí)

Characters	Pinyin	English
使道	*shǐ dào*	The pathways of the *shén qì* as in the *Elementary Questions*, Treatise 8: 使道闭塞而不通 *Shǐ dào bì sè ér bù tōng* ('The *shén* pathways are obstructed and impassable') Same as 神使之道 *shén shǐ zhī dào* (*shén* pathways)
疏泄	*shū xiè*	Course and discharge, dredge and secrete, a function of the liver *zàng* system
素问	*Sù wèn*	The *Elementary Questions,* the first part of the *Inner Canon* (*c.* 100 BCE)
素问·生气通天论	*Sù wèn, Shēng qì tōng tiān lùn*	*Elementary Questions,* 'On How the Generative [Life] *Qì* Communicates with Heaven/Nature' (Treatise 3)
素问·金匮真言论篇	*Sù wèn, Jīn guì zhēn yán lùn piān*	*Elementary Questions,* 'On the True Words in the Golden Cabinet' (Treatise 4)
素问·阴阳应象大论	*Sù wèn, Yīn yáng yīng xiàng dà lùn*	*Elementary Questions,* 'Comprehensive Discourse on Phenomena Corresponding to *Yīn* and *Yáng*' (Treatise 5)
素问·灵兰秘典论篇	*Sù wèn, Líng lán mì diǎn lùn piān*	*Elementary Questions,* 'The Secret Treatise of the Royal Library' (Treatise 8)
素问·移精变气论篇	*Sù wèn, Yí jīng biàn qì lùn piān*	*Elementary Questions,* 'On Moving the Essence and Changing the *Qì*' (Treatise 13)
素问·脉要精微论篇	*Sù wèn, Mài yào jīng wēi lùn piān*	*Elementary Questions,* 'On the Essential and Finely Discernible Aspects of the Pulse' (Treatise 17)
素问·经脉别论篇	*Sù wèn, Jīng mài bié lùn piān*	*Elementary Questions,* 'Further Discussion on the Channels and Vessels' (Treatise 21)
素问·五常政大论	*Sù wèn, Wǔ cháng zhèng dà lùn*	*Elementary Questions,* 'Great Treatise on the Five Regular Orders' (Treatise 70)
素问·刺法论篇	*Sù wèn, Cì fǎ lùn piān*	*Elementary Questions,* 'Treatise on Acupuncture Methods' (Treatise 72)

cont.

Characters	Pinyin	English
孫思邈	Sūn Sīmiǎo	581–682, author of the *Priceless and Essential Formulas for Emergencies*
太极	*tài jí*	The one, the great ultimate A state of undifferentiated and infinite potential from which *yīn* and *yáng* arise
太素	*Tài Sù (Huáng Dì nèi jíng, Tài sù)*	*Grand Basis* (*Yellow Emperor's Inner Canon, Grand Basis*), thought to have been compiled by Yáng Shàngshàn (楊上善), *c.* 656 or later, from fragments of one or several post-Han versions of the *Inner Canon* The *Tài sù* is one of four known versions of the *Inner Canon*, the other three being the *Elementary Questions*, the *Divine Pivot*, and the partially extant *Hall of Light* (明堂 *Míng táng*)
太乙金華宗旨	*Tài yǐ jīn huá zōng zhǐ*	*Secret of the Golden Flower*, said to be from the Tang dynasty, *c.* 800 CE, first published around 1680
痰蒙心窍	*tán méng xīn qiào*	Phlegm obscures (covers, dims or blinds) the heart aperture, an illness pattern (See *méng mèi* above in the entry *méng*)
痰迷心窍	*tán mí xīn qiào*	Phlegm blocks the heart aperture
天才	*tiān cái*	Genius, talent, the powers and special talents of gifted people
天神	*tiān shén*	Nature, the power of nature 'heavenly consciousness,' the 'celestial mind'—a term from the *Secret of the Golden Flower*
天性	*tiān xìng*	(A thing's inner) nature, natural instincts
王肯堂	*Wáng Kěntáng*	1549–1613, author of *Standards of Patterns and Treatments*, established the mind illness category, *shén zhì bìng*
王清任	*Wáng Qīngrèn*	1768–1831, author of *Correcting the Errors in the Forrest of Medicine* (1830)
无为	*wú wéi*	Perfect action, purposelessness, spontaneous action; non-utilitarian aim of the actions of human beings
五官	*wǔ guān*	Five offices or five officials, meaning the five senses
五神	*wǔ shén*	The five postnatal *shén* (also called 五藏神 *wǔ zàng shén*)—the 神 *shén*, 魂 *hún*, 魄 *pò*, 意 *yì* and 志 *zhì*
五体	*wǔ tǐ*	Five (body) tissues—the vessels, sinews, skin, flesh and bones

Characters	Pinyin	English
五行	*wǔ xíng*	Five phases, five transformative phases, five stages of change, five agents, five elements—wood, fire, earth, metal and water An early conceptual model describing categories of *qì* quality, relationship, movement and transformation
五运六气	*wǔ yùn liù qì*	The *Inner Canon*'s five circulatory phases and six climatic influences
五脏 (五藏)	*wǔ zàng*	The five *yīn* visceral systems—the heart, spleen, lung, kidney and liver Normally the character for *zàng* is 脏 (simplified) or 臟 (complex) In the *Inner Canon*, the *zàng*, the *yīn* visceral systems, are written 藏, without the flesh radical 月 We use 藏 for our discussions in this book because the original character is more suitable to the topic of the *shén* and its activities; 脏/臟 is more appropriate for the visceral systems and their physical–physiological activities
先天	*xiān tiān*	Prenatal, pre-heavenly, inherited, innate, ancestral, before birth
先天之先天	*xiān tiān zhī xiān tiān*	The prenatal part of the prenatal *shén* (before the foetus forms)
先天之后天	*xiān tiān zhī hòu tiān*	The prenatal part of the postnatal *shén* (after the foetus forms)
消渴	*xiāo kě*	Consumption thirst, dispersion thirst Diabetes
邪	*xié*	Evil, abnormal, intruder, askew In the medical context, *xié*-evil is a pathogen, a pathogenic influence or factor
心	*xīn*	Heart—the *zàng* of the fire phase In early Chinese texts *xīn* means the heart-mind
心窍	*xīn qiào*	Heart-*shén* aperture, specifically this is the tongue (the moving part of the voice), and more broadly the *xīn shén qiào* includes all the body openings and pores of the skin

cont.

Characters	Pinyin	English
心有所喜，神有所恶。《灵枢·大惑论》	*Xīn yǒu suǒ xǐ, shén yǒu suǒ è*	'The heart(-*shén*) loves some things and the (heart-)*shén* detests others' (from the *Divine Pivot*, Treatise 80)
心理学	*xīnlǐ xué*	(Western) psychology
心理思想	*xīnlǐ sīxiǎng*	Psychological thought A broad term for early Chinese conceptions of human mentality
新熏	*xīn xūn*	Literally, new and postnatal 'steaming–smoking' referring to acquired psychological tendencies Developmental and lifetime influences are termed 'diffuse,' meaning acquired over time with practice and habit
性	*xìng*	Nature, as in 'human nature' Basic nature, inner nature, disposition
形	*xíng*	(Body) form, shape
形神	*xíng shén*	Body form and *shén*
修身	*xiū shēn*	Self-cultivation, refinement or cultivation of the self Similar to 养生 *yǎng shēng* 'cultivating life'
修习	*xiū xí*	*Xiū*—repair, correct *Xí*—practice, habit
虚	*xū*	Depletion, deficiency, vacuity, weakness, insufficiency, emptiness
虚劳	*xū láo*	Depletion taxation, depletion wasting, vacuity taxation An illness category marked by severe depletion, weakness, fatigue and debility
熏习	*xūn xí*	*Xūn*—gradual ('smoking') practices and influences *Xí*—learn, habituate
熏染	*xūn rǎn*	Literally, 'smoking and dyeing'—*xūn rǎn* meaning gradual and sudden changes, respectively An expression for gradual and immediate influences on and changes in human psychology and personality
眼神	*yǎn shén*	The expression in the eyes, the light in a person's eyes
荀子	Xún Zǐ	*c.* 312–230 BCE, Warring States period Confucian philosopher
养生	*yǎng shēng*	Healthcare, cultivating life, self-cultivation

Characters	Pinyin	English
叶落归根	*yè luò guī gēn*	'A fallen leaf returns to its roots' (Chinese saying)
易经	*Yì jīng*	*Book of Changes*, from *c*. 700 BCE It is said that Fú Xī (伏羲 *c*. 3000 BCE, one of China's legendary chieftains) and Wén Wáng (文王 1099–1050 BCE, the founder of the Zhou dynasty 1046–221 BCE) were among its authors
义 (義)	*yì*	Dutifulness, righteousness
意	*yì*	Ideation and consciousness, one of the five postnatal *shén*, lodges in the spleen *zàng*
意识, 无意识	*yì shí,* *wú yì shí*	Conscious mind, and unconscious mind *Yìshí* is conscious reflection and ideas The processes of cognitive analysis, ideation, understanding 潜意识 *Qián yì shí* is the modern Chinese term for Western psychology's unconscious mind
抑郁	*yì yù*	Clinical depression
营气	*yíng qì*	Nutritive *qì*, construction *qì* The *yīn* partner of the 卫气 *wèi qì*-defense *qì*
忧郁	*yōu yù*	Sadness and melancholy
郁证	*yù zhèng*	Constraint pattern, binding depression pattern After the Qing dynasty, *yù zhèng* primarily refers to mental–emotional illnesses due to liver *qì* constraint
瘀	*yū*	Static blood—a pathological product
瘀阻心窍	*yū zǔ xīn qiào*	Static blood blocks the heart aperture
元	*yuán*	Initiating, primary, origin, first cause The start or beginning
元精	*yuán jīng*	Initiating (inherited, prenatal, primary, original) essence
元神	*yuán shén*	Initiating (inherited, primary, original) *shén*; the beginning of life
原	*yuán*	Source, the first unfolding
原气	*yuán qì*	Source *qì*, arises from the kidney-lifegate and distributed by the *sān jiāo*
原神	*yuán shén*	Source *shén*, the source of the postnatal *shén* An alternative name for the root *shén* (本神 *běn shén*)
岳美中	Yuè Měizhōng	1900–1982, distinguished clinician, reformer and modernizer of Chinese medicine

cont.

Characters	Pinyin	English
运化	*yùn huà*	(Spleen) transportation and transformation
脏 臟 藏	*zàng*	The *yīn* visceral system/s Literally, a coffer where treasures are stored In the *Inner Canon*, the original character is 藏 *zàng*, without the flesh radical (月)
脏腑 藏府	*zàng fǔ*	Viscera and bowels, the solid (*yīn*) and hollow (*yáng*) visceral systems of the chest and abdomen
脏躁 藏躁	*zàng zào*	Visceral agitation The name of an emotion-related illness that first appeared in Zhāng Zhòngjǐng's *Golden Cabinet* (*c.* 200 CE)
张从正	Zhāng Cóngzhèng	1156–1228, author of the *Confucians' Duties to Their Parents* (儒门事亲 *Rú mén shì qīn*)
张仲景	Zhāng Zhòngjǐng	150–219 CE, author of the *Treatise on Cold Damage and Miscellaneous Disorders* (伤寒杂病论 *Shānghán zábìng lùn*) *c.* 220 Nowadays this is two books: *On Cold Damage* and *Essential Prescriptions of the Golden Cabinet*
真君子	*zhēn jūn zǐ*	The ideal of a 'true gentleman,' a wise, ethical, exemplary person
正	*zhèng*	Correct, upright *Zhèng qì* is the opposite of *xié*-evil *qì*
智	*zhì*	Intelligence, moral intelligence
智慧	*zhì huì*	Wisdom
志	*zhì*	Mind, memory, will, determination, ambition, intelligence Emotion, temperament, disposition The *zhì* is one of the five postnatal *shén*, it resides in the kidney *zàng*
滞	*zhì*	Stagnation, the inhibited movement of *qì* or food, as in, for example, 'liver *qì* stagnation'
中根	*zhōng gēn*	The central root, the inner root The foundation that generates *qì* in all phenomena A thing's natural disposition
主	*zhǔ*	Ruler–host, lord, governor

Characters	Pinyin	English
祝由	*zhù yóu*	Announcing causes A pre-modern therapeutic strategy whereby the doctor would determine the root of their patient's illness and make this known to them—announcing causes was believed to assist patients in changing their view of themselves
朱丹溪	Zhū Dānxī	1281–1358, Yuan scholar–physician (also known as 朱震亨 Zhū Zhènhēng)
自然	*zì rán*	What is so of itself Spontaneously self-generating Nature
宗教	*zōng jiào*	Religion
做梦	*zuò mèng*	Dream, (normal nighttime) dreaming

References and Further Reading

Ames, R.T. (1993) 'The Meaning of Body in Classical Chinese Philosophy.' In T.P. Kasulis, *Self as Body in Asian Theory and Practice*, pp.157–177. Albany, NY: State University of New York Press.

Birch, S., Cabrer Mir, M.A. and Cuadras, M.R. (2014) *Restoring Order in Health and Chinese Medicine: Studies of the Development and Use of Qì and the Channels.* Barcelona: La Liebre de Marzo.

Bromley, M., Freeman, D., Hext, A. and Rochat de la Vallee, E. (2010) *Jing Shen: A Translation of Huainanzi Chapter Seven.* London: Monkey Press.

Chace, C. and Bensky, D. (2009) 'An axis of efficacy: The range of meaning in the *Ling Shu* Chapter One, Part 1.' *The Lantern*, 6(1): 5–13.

Chen, H.F. (2014) 'Emotional Therapy and Talking Cures in Late Imperial China.' In H. Chiang, *Psychiatry and Chinese History*, pp.37–54. London: Pickering and Chatto.

Chiang, H. (ed.) (2014) *Psychiatry and Chinese History.* London: Pickering and Chatto.

Chiu, M.L. (1986) *Mind, Body, and Illness in a Chinese Medical Tradition.* Doctor of Philosophy in History and East Asian Languages, Harvard University.

Christians, J.K. and Keightley, P.D. (2005) 'Behavioural genetics: Finding genes that cause complex trait variation.' *Current Biology*, 15(1): R19–R21.

Cleary, T. (1981) *The Secret of the Golden Flower: The Classic Chinese Book of Life.* New York, NY: HarperOne.

Cosmides, L. and Tooby, J. (1997) 'Evolutionary Psychology: A Primer.' Available at www.psych.ucsb.edu/research/cep/primer.html.

Deadman, P., Al-Khafaji, M. and Baker, K. (1998) *A Manual of Acupuncture.* Hove: Journal of Chinese Medicine Publications.

Farquhar, J. (1994) *Knowing Practice: The Clinical Encounter of Chinese Medicine.* Boulder, CO: Westview Press.

Freud, S. (1977) *Case Histories I—'Dora' and 'Little Hans.'* Hammondsworth: Penguin.

Fu, Q.Z. (1996, originally 1826) *Fu Qìng-Zhu's Gynecology* (trans. S.Z. Yang and D.W. Liu). Boulder, CO: Blue Poppy Press.

Fuller, J.L. and Thompson, W.R. (1964) *Behavior Genetics*. New York, NY: John Wiley and Sons.

Garvey, M. (2001) 'Hysteria.' *Clinical Acupuncture and Oriental Medicine*, 2(4): 221–227.

Garvey, M. (2015) *A Clinical Guide to the Body in Chinese Medicine: History and Contemporary Practice*. Taos, NM: Paradigm Publications.

Garvey, M. and Qu, L.F. (2001) 'The liver's shuxie function.' *European Journal of Oriental Medicine*, 3(5): 32–37.

Geaney, J. (2002) *On the Epistemology of the Senses in Early Chinese Thought*. Honolulu: University of Hawai'i Press.

Hou, J. (1996) *Traditional Chinese Treatment for Psychogenic and Neurogenic Diseases*. Beijing: Academy Press.

Huang, F.M. (1994) *Jia Yi Jing, The Systematic Classic of Acupuncture and Moxibustion* (trans. S.Z. Yang and C. Chace). Boulder, CO: Blue Poppy Press.

Jung, C.G. (1980) 'Foreword,' third English edition. In R. Wilhelm, *The I Ching, or Book of Changes*, pp.xxi–xxxix. London: Routledge and Kegan Paul.

Jung, C.G. (1984) 'Foreword,' second German edition. In R. Wilhelm, *The Secret of the Golden Flower: A Chinese Book of Life*, pp. xiii–xv. London: Arkana.

Kohn, L. (1992) *Early Chinese Mysticism: Philosophy and Soteriology in the Taoist Tradition*. Princeton, NJ: Princeton University Press.

Kuriyama, S. (1999) *The Expressiveness of the Body and the Divergence of Greek and Chinese Medicine*. New York, NY: Zone Books.

Lai, K. (2006) *Learning from Chinese Philosophies: Ethics of Interdependent and Contextualised Self*. Aldershot, Hampshire: Ashgate Publishing.

Larre, C. and Rochat de La Vallee, E. (1992) *The Secret Treatise of the Spiritual Orchid: Neijing Suwen Chapter 8*. Cambridge: Monkey Press.

Lloyd, G. and Sivin, N. (2002) *The Way and The Word: Science and Medicine in Early China and Greece*. New York, NY: Yale University Press.

Lo, V. (2001) 'The Influence of Nurturing Life Culture on the Development of Western Han Acumoxa Therapy.' In E. Hsu, *Innovation in Chinese Medicine*, pp.19–50. Cambridge: Cambridge University Press.

May, B.H., Feng, M., Zhou, I.W., Chang, S.-y. *et al.* (2016) 'Memory impairment, dementia, and Alzheimer's disease in classical and contemporary Traditional Chinese Medicine.' *Journal of Alternative and Complementary Medicine*, 22(9): 695–705.

Nairne, J.S. and Pandeirada, J.N.S. (2010) 'Adaptive memory: Ancestral priorities and the mnemonic value of survival processing.' *Cognitive Psychology*, 61(1): 1–22.

Nivison, D.S. (1999) 'The Classical Philosophical Writings.' In M. Loewe and E.L. Shaughnessy, *The Cambridge History of Ancient China: From the Origins of Civilization to 221 B.C.*, pp.745–884. Cambridge: Cambridge University Press.

Porkert, M. (1979) *The Theoretical Foundations of Chinese Medicine: Systems of Correspondence*. Cambridge, MA: MIT Press.

Qian, B.X. (2006) *Qian Boxuan Case Studies in Gynecology*. Beijing: People's Medical Publishing House.

Qu, L.F. (2015) *Mental and Psychological Diseases: Selected Cases of Ancient Masters*. Shanghai: Science and Technology Press (in Chinese: 曲丽芳 2013 精神心理疾病: 历代名家验案选粹, 上海科学出版社).

Qu, L.F. and Garvey, M. (2006) 'Shen-zhi theory: Analysis of the signs and symptoms of mental disorder.' *European Journal of Oriental Medicine*, 5(2): 4–17.

Qu, L.F. and Garvey, M. (2008) 'Exploring the difference between Chinese medicine and biomedicine using the *Yi Jing*'s epistemic methodology.' *Australian Journal of Acupuncture and Chinese Medicine*, 3(1): 17–24.

Qu, L.F. and Garvey, M. (2009a) 'The psychological significance of Yuanshen and Shishen.' *The Journal of Chinese Medicine*, 91: 61–67.

Qu, L.F. and Garvey, M. (2009b) 'On the psychological significance of heart governing *Shen Ming*.' *Australian Journal of Acupuncture and Chinese Medicine*, 4(1): 14–22.

Qu, L.F. and M. Garvey (2016) *Anecdotes of Traditional Chinese Medicine: A Bilingual Extracurricular Reader for Traditional Chinese Medicine*. Shanghai: Shanghai Science and Technology Press. Re-released (2018) by the World Century Publishing Corporation, Singapore.

Qu, L.F. and Zhang, W.H. (2015) *Psychiatry of Chinese Medicine*. Shanghai: Science and Technology Press (in Chinese: 曲丽芳, 张苇航 2015 中医神志病学. 上海科学出版社).

Rossi, E. (2007) *Shen: Psycho-Emotional Aspects of Chinese Medicine*. London: Churchill Livingstone.

Roth, H.D. (1991) 'Psychology and self-cultivation in early Taoistic thought.' *Harvard Journal of Asiatic Studies*, 51(2): 599–650.

Scheid, V. (2007) *Currents of Tradition in Chinese Medicine 1626–2006*. Seattle, WA: Eastland Press.

Scheid, V. (2013) 'Depression, constraint, and the liver: (Dis)assembling the treatment of emotion-related disorders in Chinese medicine.' *Culture, Medicine and Psychiatry*, 37(1): 30–58.

Simonis, F. (2014) 'Medicaments and Persuasion: Medical Therapies for Madness in Nineteenth-Century China.' In H. Chiang (ed.), *Psychiatry and Chinese History*, pp.55–70. London: Pickering and Chatto.

Sivin, N. (1987) *Traditional Medicine in Contemporary China: A Partial Translation of Revised Outline of Chinese Medicine (1972): With an Introductory Study on Change in Present Day and Early Medicine*. Ann Arbor, MI: Center for Chinese Studies, University of Michigan.

Sung, B. (1990) *Classical Moxibustion Skills in Contemporary Clinical Practice*. Boulder, CO: Blue Poppy Press.

[Unknown] (1999/*c.* 8th century) *The Yellow Emperor's Hidden Talisman Canon*. 黄帝阴符经集注. Z. Zhou and B. Chang. Beijing: Chinese Drama Press.

Unschuld, P.U. (1986) *The Chinese Medical Classics: Nan-Ching, The Classic of Difficult Issues*. Berkeley, CA: University of California Press.

Unschuld, P.U. (2009) *What Is Medicine? Western and Eastern Approaches to Healing*. Berkeley, CA: University of California Press.

Unschuld, P.U. and Tessenow, H. (2011) *Huangdi Neijing Suwen*. Berkeley, CA: University of California Press.

Vance, B.E. (2014). 'Exorcising Dreams and Nightmares in Late Ming China.' In H. Chiang, *Psychiatry and Chinese History*, pp.17–36. London: Pickering and Chatto.

Wieger, L. (1965) *Chinese Characters: Their Origin, Etymology, History, Classification and Signification. A Thorough Study from Chinese Documents*. New York, NY: Paragon Book Reprint Corp.

Wilhelm, R. (1984) *The Secret of the Golden Flower: A Chinese Book of Life*. London: Arkana.

Wilms, S. (2002) 'The Female Body in Medieval China: A Translation and Interpretation of the "Women's Recipes".' In Sŭn Sīmiăo, *Beiji Qìanjin Yaofang*. Tucson, AZ: The University of Arizona.

Wiseman, N., Wilms, S. and Zhang, Z.J. (2013) *Jin Gui Yao Lue: Essential Prescriptions of the Golden Cabinet, Translation and Commentaries*. Taos, NM: Paradigm Publications.

Xiong J. (Hunan College of Traditional Chinese Medicine) (1981) 'A case using Zhusha Anshen Pill and Magnetic Zhu Wan to cure night wandering syndrome.' *Journal of Chinese Medicine*, 11, p.62 熊继柏 (湖南中医学院内经教研室), '朱砂安神丸合磁朱丸治愈夜游症1 例', 中医杂志, 62 (In Chinese, available from the China Academic Journal Electronic Publishing House, www.cnki.net).

Yan, S.L. and Li, Z.H. (2007) *Pathomechanisms of the Liver: Gan Bing Zhi Bing Ji*. Taos, NM: Paradigm Publications.

Yates, R.D.S. (1994) 'Body, Space, Time and Bureaucracy: Boundary Creation and Control Mechanisms in Early China.' In J. Hay, *Boundaries in China*, pp.56–80. London: Reaktion Books.

Yuè, M.Z. (2007) *Yuè MěiZhōng Collected Case Studies*. Beijing: People's Medical Publishing House.

Zhang, D.N. (2002) *Key Concepts in Chinese Philosophy*. Beijing: Foreign Languages Press.

Zhang, Y.H. (2007) *Transforming Emotions with Chinese Medicine: An Ethnographic Account from Contemporary China*. New York, NY: State University of New York Press.

Index

acquired *shén* 14, 15, 66–7
acupuncture points
  agitation 210
  anger 210
  anxiety 210
  dementia 210
  depletion taxation 210
  depression 211
  dreams 211
  fearfulness 211
  forgetfulness 211
  insomnia 211
  lily disease 211
  mania 211
  manic depression 211
  menopausal syndrome 211
  palpitation (from fright) 212
  plum pit *qì* (globus hystericus) 212
  postpartum exhaustion 212
  psychosis 212
  running piglet *qì* disease 212
  sadness 212
  sea of marrow 212
  thinking 212
  vexation 212
  visceral agitation 212
  worry 212
ADHD 103
adrenal response 61
agitation (acupuncture points) 210
  see also visceral agitation
Ames, R.T. 39

ancestral/evolutionary information 56–8
anger, acupuncture points 210
announcing causes 32
anxiety
  acupuncture points 210
  bupleurum plus dragon bone and
    oyster shell decoction 174
  escape restraint pill 146–7
  flush the phlegm decoction 182
  free wanderer powder 148
  fried liquorice decoction 178–9
  Heavenly Emperor's tonify
    the heart pill 137
  lily combination 132
  liquorice, wheat and jujube
    decoction 135
  overview 177
  pinellia and magnolia bark
    decoction 133–4
  restore the spleen decoction 139
  running piglet decoction 141–2
  settle the emotions pill 138, 169–70
  seven blessings decoction 183–4
  spiny jujube decoction 168
  true warrior decoction 179
  warm the gallbladder decoction 175
archetypes 57, 114–5
astragalus and cinnamon twig five
  substance decoction 163
autism spectrum disorder 104
awaken from the nightmare of
  madness decoction 176

Běn shén (root shén) 14, 21, 55–8
bēn tún qì-running piglet qì 197–9
Bing, Wáng 43
body–mind, in Chinese medicine 37–8
Book of Changes 13, 18, 19, 20, 96
brain essence and shén míng 93–5
Breuer, J. 114, 116
Bromley, M. 120
Buddhism 96–7
bupleurum plus dragon bone and
    oyster shell decoction 174
bupleurum powder to dredge
    the liver 153–4

Canon of Difficult Issues 26
cases
    ben tun qì-running piglet qì 197–9
    depressive psychosis 204–6
    excess joy causing kuáng-
        madness 189–90
    fear overcomes excess joy 188
    hún wandering 190–1
    hún–pò wandering 191–5
    joy therapy 186–7
    mania for seven years after
        thwarted ambition 201–4
    menopausal syndrome 196–7
    panic attacks 197–9
    postpartum depressive
        psychosis 206–7
    shén–hún disharmony 190–1
    thinking 185
    turbid phlegm fire leading
        to insanity 199–201
    zàng zao-visceral agitation 196–7
Changes, The 20
Chen, H.F. 30, 32
Chén Xiūyuán 191
Chén Yán 146, 147, 175
Chiang, H. 32
children, formulas for use
    with 135, 143, 145, 174
Chinese angelica and peony powder 158
Chiu, M.L. 30, 37
Christians, J.K. 114
cinnamon twig plus dragon bone and
    oyster shell decoction 143, 164
Classified Classic 29
cleanse the heart decoction 181

Cleary, T. 46, 47, 54
collective unconscious 114–5
conception, moment of 18, 36, 49, 54
Confucianism 96
conscious awareness
    in psychoanalytical theory 114–6
    in tree of human life analogy 118–9
constitution 83–6
constraint syndrome 146–51
correct qì 95
Cosmides, L. 114

dang gui center-fortifying
    decoction 161–2
Dào dé jing 18
Daoism 96
dào–phenomenon–entity triad 19
defense mechanisms 117
dementia
    acupuncture points 210
    bupleurum plus dragon bone and
        oyster shell decoction 174
    Chinese angelica and
        peony powder 158
    cleanse the heart decoction 181
    eight-ingredient kidney qì pill 156
    flush the phlegm decoction 103, 182
    major bupleurum decoction 172–3
    open the apertures and quicken
        the blood decoction 182–3
    overview 180–1
    right restoring pill 155
    seven blessings decoction 183–4
    warm the gallbladder decoction 175
depletion taxation
    acupuncture points 210
    cinnamon twig plus dragon bone
        and oyster shell decoction 143
    minor center-fortifying decoction 145
    overview 142–4
depression
    acupuncture points 211
    astragalus and cinnamon twig
        five substance decoction 163
    awaken from the nightmare of
        madness decoction 176
    bupleurum plus dragon bone and
        oyster shell decoction 174

bupleurum powder to dredge
    the liver 153–4
Chinese angelica and
    peony powder 158
cinnamon twig plus dragon bone
    and oyster shell decoction 143
dang gui center-fortifying
    decoction 161–2
drive out stasis in the mansion
    of blood decoction 170–1
eight-ingredient kidney *qì* pill 156
escape restraint pill 146–7, 152–3
flush the phlegm decoction 182
free wanderer powder 148, 153
frigid extremities powder 149, 153
lily combination 132
liquorice, wheat and jujube
    decoction 135
liver stagnation and constraint
    treatments 152–4
major bupleurum decoction 172–3
minor bupleurum decoction 160–1
minor center-fortifying decoction 145
open the apertures and quicken
    the blood decoction 182–3
pinellia and magnolia bark
    decoction 133–4
restore the spleen decoction 139
right restoring pill 155
running piglet decoction 141–2
settle the emotions pill 138, 169–70
warm the gallbladder decoction 175
depressive psychosis (case study) 204–6
developmental stages 62–5
diagnosis, in Chinese
    psychological thought 30
Divine Pivot
    Treatise 8 35–7, 55
    Treatise 43 110, 129–30
    Treatise 64 84
dreams
    acupuncture points 211
    connecting inner and outer world 108
    disturbing 130
    Forest of Dreams 108–9
    Inner Canon on 110–2
    mechanisms of 109
    nightmares 108, 138, 143, 191–3
    research into 107

drive out stasis in the mansion
    of blood decoction 170–1
drives 60–1

earth phase personality 85
eating disorders (minor center-
    fortifying decoction) 145
eight-ingredient kidney *qì* pill 156, 166
Elementary Questions
    Treatise 8 34–5, 89–90, 91
    Treatise 13 55
    Treatise 21 93–4
    Treatise 70 40
    Treatise 72 98
    Treatise 80 110
emotional catharsis therapy 31–2
emotions, effects of 24, 27, 77–8
epilepsy (bupleurum plus dragon bone
    and oyster shell decoction) 174
escape restraint pill 146–7
essence (brain) 93–5
essence *shén* 49–50
*Essential Prescriptions of the Golden
    Cabinet* 26, 123–4, 131, 157, 159
ethical conduct 95–101
'evil crying' 26
'evil *qì*' 95
evolution of human life 56–8, 114
evolutionary psychology 114
excess joy causing *kuáng*-madness
    (case study) 189–90

Farquhar, J. 30
fear overcomes excess joy
    (case study) 188
fearfulness
    acupuncture points 211
    bupleurum plus dragon bone and
        oyster shell decoction 174
    cinnamon twig plus dragon bone
        and oyster shell decoction 143
    restore the spleen decoction 139
    running piglet decoction 141–2
    settle the emotions pill 138
Fèi Bóxióng *199*, 200
fire phase personality 85
five phases (*Inner Canon*) 31, 85
five *shén* theory 74–6

five *zàng shén* 36, 38, 66–7
flush the phlegm decoction 182
foetal development 58
food/nourishment 93–4
forgetfulness
    acupuncture points 211
    cinnamon twig plus dragon bone
        and oyster shell decoction 143
    cleanse the heart decoction 181
    drive out stasis in the mansion
        of blood decoction 170–1
    eight-ingredient kidney *qì* pill 156
    fried liquorice decoction 178–9
    Heavenly Emperor's tonify
        the heart pill 137
    restore the spleen decoction 139
    right restoring pill 155
    settle the emotions pill 138, 169–70
    seven blessings decoction 183–4
    spiny jujube decoction 168
    true warrior decoction 179
free wanderer powder 148, 165–6
Freud, S. 114, 116–7, 136
fried liquorice decoction 178–9
frigid extremities powder 149
Fù Qīngzhu 162, 163
Fu, Q.Z. 162
Fuller, J.L. 114

Garvey, M. 20, 32, 55, 66,
    101, 116, 128, 136, 151
Geaney, J. 21, 101
globus hystericus *see* plum pit
    qì (globus hystericus)
Golden Flower text 54, 59
gynecological pain 157–8

hallucinations 27–9, 175
heart
    pictographs/character 23
    in *shén zhì* theory 73, 75
heart-mind 22–3
heart-*shén* (sovereign ruler)
    cultivating brightness 91–2, 95–101
    inter-relationships 79–80
    overview 34, 38, 68–9
    without clarity and brightness 101–4
Heavenly Emperor's tonify
    the heart pill 137, 165

hepatitis
    bupleurum powder to dredge
        the liver 153–4
    frigid extremities powder 149
Hidden Talisman Canon 54
history *see* psychological
    thought (Chinese)
Hou, J. 103
Huá Tuó 31
Huáng Dì 28
human life
    basis of 39–46
    as divine 48
    origin of 46–51
    prenatal and postnatal 61
human nature, in Chinese
    psychological thought 20–1
hún wandering 190–1
hún–pò wandering 129–30, 191–5

iceberg analogy 115–6
initiating *shén* 14–5, 58–66
Inner Canon 13–4, 18, 24,
    25, 33, 50, 110–2
inner root 42–3, 50–1
insomnia
    acupuncture points 211
    astragalus and cinnamon twig
        five substance decoction 163
    bupleurum plus dragon bone and
        oyster shell decoction 174
    bupleurum powder to dredge
        the liver 153–4
    cinnamon twig plus dragon bone
        and oyster shell decoction 143
    dang gui center-fortifying
        decoction 161–2
    drive out stasis in the mansion
        of blood decoction 170–1
    free wanderer powder 148
    fried liquorice decoction 178–9
    Heavenly Emperor's tonify
        the heart pill 137
    lily combination 132
    liquorice, wheat and jujube
        decoction 135
    major bupleurum decoction 172–3
    major order the *qì* decoction 159
    minor center-fortifying decoction 145

open the apertures and quicken
  the blood decoction 182–3
overview 166
peach pit order the *qì* decoction 160
pinellia and magnolia bark
  decoction 133–4
pinellia and millet decoction 166–7
psychosis, minor bupleurum
  decoction 160–1
restore the spleen decoction 139
settle the emotions pill 138, 169–70
seven blessings decoction 183–4
spiny jujube decoction 168
true warrior decoction 179
warm the gallbladder decoction 175
instincts 60–1
inter-relationships, complex 79–83

jing shén 24–5, 58
joy therapy 186–7
Jung, C.G. 57, 114, 115

Keightley, P.D. 114
kidney, in *shén zhì* theory 73, 76, 80
kidney illness patterns 156
Kohn, L. 37

Lai, K. 47
Lǐ Shízhēn 59
Lǐ Tǐng 27
Li, Z.H. 151
lily bulb disease
  acupuncture points 211
  treatment 129, 131–3
lily combination 132, 157, 164
liquorice, wheat and jujube
  decoction 135, 157, 165
Líu Wánsù 27
liver, in *shén zhì* theory 73, 75, 81
Lloyd, G. 12
lung, in *shén zhì* theory 73, 75, 82

major order the *qì* decoction 159
mania
  acupuncture points 211
  awaken from the nightmare of
    madness decoction 176
bupleurum plus dragon bone and
  oyster shell decoction 174
in Chinese psychological
  thought 25–6
major bupleurum decoction 172–3
major order the *qì* decoction 159
peach pit order the *qì* decoction 160
settle the emotions pill 170
mania for seven years after thwarted
  ambition (case study) 201–4
manic depression, acupuncture
  points 211
memory *see* forgetfulness
Mèng Zǐ
  39, 92, 96
menopausal syndrome
  acupuncture points 211
  bupleurum plus dragon bone and
    oyster shell decoction 174
  case study 197
  Chinese angelica and
    peony powder 158
  cinnamon twig plus dragon bone and
    oyster shell decoction 143, 164
  drive out stasis in the mansion
    of blood decoction 170–1
  eight-ingredient kidney
    qì pill 156, 166
  free wanderer powder 148, 165–6
  Heavenly Emperor's tonify
    the heart pill 137, 165
  lily combination 132, 157, 164
  liquorice, wheat and jujube
    decoction 135, 165
  minor bupleurum decoction 165
  overview 164
  peach pit order the *qì* decoction 160
  pinellia and magnolia bark
    decoction 133–4, 164
  psychosis, minor bupleurum
    decoction 160–1
  right restoring pill 155
  spiny jujube decoction 166, 168
  warm the gallbladder decoction 175
menstrual disorders
  bupleurum powder to dredge
    the liver 153–4
  free wanderer powder 148
mental capacity deterioration 101–4
metal phase personality 85

'mind' *see shén*
'mind category' 29–30
mìng mén 62
minor bupleurum decoction 160–1, 165
minor center-fortifying decoction 145
monism 13
Mòzǐ 39

Nairne, J.S. 114
nature, power of 46–7
'neurosis' 117
nightmares 108, 138, 143, 191–3
Nivison, D.S. 92
nourishment/food 93–4

open the apertures and quicken
    the blood decoction 182–3
over-eating 94

palpitation from fright
    acupuncture points 212
Pandeirada, J.N.S. 114
panic attacks 197–9
peach pit order the *qì* decoction 160
personality
    five phase types (*Inner Canon*) 85
    influences on 117–8
    shǎoyáng types 84
    shǎoyin types 83–4
    tàiyáng types 84
    tàiyīn types 83
phlegm misting the heart aperture 102–4
phobias
    cinnamon twig plus dragon bone
        and oyster shell decoction 143
    running piglet decoction 141–2
pinellia and magnolia bark
    decoction 133–4, 164
pinellia and millet decoction 166–7
plum pit *qì*, escape restraint pill 146–7
plum pit *qì* (globus hystericus) 133–4
    acupuncture points 212
Porkert, M. 91
possession 25–7
postnatal life 61–5
postpartum depression and psychosis
    astragalus and cinnamon twig
        five substance decoction 163

case study 206–7
dang gui center-fortifying
    decoction 161–2
major order the *qì* decoction 159
minor bupleurum decoction 160–1
overview 158–9
peach pit order the *qì* decoction 160
postpartum exhaustion,
    acupuncture points 212
postpartum fever, psychosis, minor
    bupleurum decoction 160–1
power of nature 46–7
prenatal life 61–5
psychoanalytic theory 114–7
psychological thought (Chinese)
    early psychological disorders 25–30
    early treatment strategies 30–3
    human nature 20–1
    'mind category' 29–30
    overview 17–20
    shén in 21–5
psychology (Western) 113–7
psychosis
    acupuncture points 212
    awaken from the nightmare of
        madness decoction 176
    bupleurum plus dragon bone and
        oyster shell decoction 174
    bupleurum powder to dredge
        the liver 153–4
    dang gui center-fortifying
        decoction 161–2
    depressive psychosis (case
        study) 204–6
    drive out stasis in the mansion
        of blood decoction 170–1
    escape restraint pill 146–7
    liquorice, wheat and jujube
        decoction 135
    major bupleurum decoction 172–3
    major order the *qì* decoction 159
    mania for seven years after thwarted
        ambition (case) 201–4
    minor bupleurum decoction 160–1
    overview 172
    peach pit order the *qì* decoction 160
    pinellia and magnolia bark
        decoction 133–4
    running piglet decoction 141–2

spiny jujube decoction 168
warm the gallbladder decoction 175

qì, concept of 12–3
Qi Bó 206
qì set-up 45–6
Qian, B.X. 196, 197
qíng zhì theory 76–8
Qu, L.F. 10, 20, 32, 55,
    66, 101, 116, 151

relationships, complex 79–83
rén shén 48
right restoring pill 155
root *shén* 14, 21, 55–8
root-tendency psychology 119–20
Roth, Harold 17
running piglet *qì* disease
    acupuncture points 212
    overview 140–1
    running piglet decoction 141–2

sadness (acupuncture points) 212
Scheid, V. 148
sea of marrow (acupuncture points) 212
self, sense of 66
self-cultivation 97–101
sensory apertures 67–9, 100, 101–4
settle the emotions pill 138, 169–70
seven blessings decoction 183–4
shǎoyáng types 84
shǎoyin types 83–4
shén
    in Chinese psychological
        thought 21–5, 38
    influence of 14–5
    overview of three aspects 53–5
    pictographs for 22
    see also acquired *shén*;
        initiating *shén*; root *shén*
shén dynamic 43–4
shén míng (brightness)
    brain essence and 93–5
    heart-ruler cultivating 95–101
    heart-ruler with 91–2
    heart-ruler without 101–4
    overview 89–90

shén wandering 131
shén zhì bìng 128
shén zhì theory 72–6
shén–hún disharmony 128, 190–1
shén–pò disharmony 128–9
shí shén (acquired *shén*) 14, 15, 66–7
Sivin, N. 12, 30, 49
sleepwalking 130, 132, 135, 168, 193–5
spiny jujube decoction 166, 168
spleen, in *shén zhì* theory 73, 75, 80
static blood 102–4
Sūn Sīmiǎo 138, 162, 163
Sūn Zéxiān 118

tàiyáng types 84
tàiyīn types 83
'talking cure' 30–2
terminology 12, 22–5
thinking, acupuncture points 212
thinking (case study) 185
Thompson, W.R. 114
three treasures 22
tiān shén 46–7
Tooby, J. 114
tree of human life analogy 118–9
tricks, doctor playing 31–2
triple burner 62
true warrior decoction 179
turbid phlegm fire leading
    to insanity 199–201

unconscious (in psychoanalytic
    theory) 114–7
Unschuld, P.U. 47

Vance, B.E. 108, 109
vexation, acupuncture points 212
visceral agitation
    acupuncture points 212
    Heavenly Emperor's tonify
        the heart pill 137
    liquorice, wheat and jujube
        decoction 135
    overview 134–6
    restore the spleen decoction 139
    settle the emotions pill 138
    zàng zao-visceral agitation 196–7
visceral manifestations theory 20

Wáng Bīng *43*
Wáng Kìntáng 29, 76
Wáng Qīngrèn 103, 170, 176, 182
warm the gallbladder decoction 175
water phase personality 85
Wieger, L. 22, 59, 120
Wilhelm, R. 46, 54, 67, 115
Wilms, S. 162
wood phase personality 85
worry, acupuncture points 212
Wú Jutōng 32, 2301, 204

xiàng 19
Xú Dàchūn 188
Xuān Yuán 206
Xúnzǐ 92

Yan, S.L. 151
Yates, R.D.S. 92

Yè Tiānshi 150, 204
Yellow Emperor's Inner Canon
  see Inner Canon
yīn–yáng natural law 18, 19, 20, 84
Yuán shén (initiating *shén*) 14–5, 58–66
Yue, M.Z. 162, 163, 198–9

zàng fu 92
zàng shén 36, 38, 66–7
zàng zao-visceral agitation 196–7
Zhāng Cóngzhèng 31, 32, 187
Zhang, D.N. 19, 21, 47, 60
Zhāng Jièbin 19, 29, 76, 108, 156, 183
Zhang, Y.H. 77, 150
Zhāng Zhòngjǐng 26, 123, 124,
  131, 132, 133, 134, 141, 142,
  144, 148, 155, 159, 162, 179
Zhào Xiànkě 147
Zhū Dānxī 27, 146, 147, 154